Current Practice in Health Sciences Librarianship

Alison Bunting

Editor-in-Chief

Volume 5
Acquisitions in Health Sciences Libraries

Edited by
David H. Morse

Medical Library Association
and
The Scarecrow Press, Inc.
Lanham, Md. & London

British Library Cataloguing-in-Publication Information Available

Library of Congress Cataloging-in-Publication Data

Acquisitions in health sciences libraries / edited by David H. Morse.
      p. cm. — (Current practice in health sciences librarianship; v. 5)
   Includes bibliographical references and index.
   ISBN 0–8108–3052–3 (alk. paper).
   1. Medical libraries—Acquisitions—United States. I. Morse, David H.
II. Series.
Z675.M4A35   1996
26.61'0973—dc21
                                          96–46948
                                            CIP

ISBN 0–8108–3052–3 (cloth : alk. paper)

Acquisitions in
Health Sciences Libraries

Contents

Preface

Current Practice in Health Sciences Librarianship (CPHSL) continues the publication principles established by its predecessor, the *Handbook of Medical Library Practice*, to serve as: a general introduction to the field of health sciences librarianship for graduate students; a source of basic information and references to the literature for the Medical Library Association's (MLA) professional development and recognition program; a reference work for health sciences librarians and other information specialists, providing basic information in areas peripheral to their own expertise; and a means of documenting the state of practice of health sciences librarianship at a particular point in time.

The decision to change the title of this venerable MLA publication is best explained by a review of the *Handbook*'s publication history. The appearance in 1942 of the first edition of the *Handbook*, published by the American Library Association, fulfilled a long-standing goal of the MLA. As editor Janet Doe noted,

> The demand [for a Handbook] has grown keener with the passage of time, undoubtedly because of the recent rapid increase in the number of medical libraries, for half of the 315 now existing in this country have originated since 1910. To staff these libraries, workers have been enticed or commandeered from general and special libraries, from library schools, from the clerical staff of hospitals or medical schools, and from doctors' offices [1].

The second edition of the *Handbook* (1956), edited by Janet Doe and Mary Louise Marshall [2], updated the one-volume first edition, retaining, whenever possible, the original chapter authors. The preface to this volume included an apology for publication delays and noted that some of the information in the volume was written three or more years prior to publication.

Fourteen years elapsed before the third edition, the first one published by MLA, appeared in 1970. Editors Gertrude L. Annan and Jacqueline W. Felter took an entirely different approach: "The chapters are written by a new cadre of authors and differ from those of the earlier edition in substance and emphasis" [3]. Despite the expansion of the scope and coverage, the one-volume format was retained. Four consultants from different types of health sciences libraries ensured that the content took into account library practice in these settings. Publication delays continued to be a problem and were

> ...of grave concern to the editors who regret that some chapters were written several years before the volume went to press. With so many involved in the preparation of the work, unforeseen emergencies arose which prevented its production in the period scheduled [4].

Louise Darling, David Bishop, and Lois Ann Colaianni edited the fourth edition, published between 1982 and 1988. This edition included a "...shift in terminology from medical to health science libraries...in it-self...indicative of the new complexity, the highly interdisciplinary nature of the fields served by these libraries" [5]. However, the title of the *Handbook* was not changed "...because of the risk of obscuring the continuity of editions" [6]. A three-volume format was chosen to: "...accommodate material on new developments, lessen the delays inherent in a mutiple-author work, and facilitate later revision..." [7]. This new approach did not, however, prevent publication delays

> ...even with a smaller number of authors per volume, the consid-erable time difference in submission of chapters has meant that the problem of keeping material within the volume on the same level of currency, though reduced, has not been solved [8].

And, "...the sequential publication has resulted in problems of uneven currency in the completed work..." [9]. "A more satisfactory method for revising the Handbook in the future is now under study, as the rapid pace of change in the information field obviously requires a new approach" [10].

In 1989, the MLA Books Panel recommended that the *Handbook* be continued with the same general scope and content as the fourth edition, but that the three volumes be further divided into a series of smaller monographs, each dealing with a single subject and each with its own volume editor. An editor-in-chief, assisted by an Advisory Committee, was appointed to coordinate the publication.

The Advisory Committee determined that health sciences librarianship is changing so rapidly that the profession will be better served by publica-tion of a series, and that the series required a new title. In this way, individual volumes can be updated as needed, without having to wait for the completion of all volumes in an edition, and the individual volumes will have a greater identity as independent books.

CPHSL will appear in eight volumes. The editors are noted below:

Volume 1: Reference and Information Services in Health Sciences Libraries, *M. Sandra Wood, editor*

Volume 2: Educational Services in Health Sciences Libraries, *Francesca Allegri, editor*

Volume 3: Information Access and Delivery in Health Sciences Libraries, *Carolyn Lipscomb, editor*

Volume 4: Collection Development and Assessment in Health Sciences Libraries, *Daniel T. Richards and Dottie Eakin*

Volume 5: Acquisitions in Health Sciences Libraries, *David H. Morse, editor*

Volume 6: Bibliographic Management of Information Resources in Health Sciences Libraries, *Laurie L. Thompson, editor*

Volume 7: Health Sciences Environment and Librarianship in Health Sciences Libraries, *Lucretia W. McClure, editor*

Volume 8: Administration and Management in Health Sciences Libraries, *Rick B. Forsman, editor*

The editor-in-chief is extremely fortunate in being able to tap the expertise of a group of very talented and dedicated MLA members as advisors, editors, and chapter authors. The CPHSL Advisory Committee provided valuable advice on the organization and content of CPHSL, recommended a publication plan and timetable, and assisted in the identification of editors and chapter authors.

The editors have total responsibility for the preparation for publication of their volume, including selection of authors, review of content and adherence to established style and format guidelines, and maintenance of the publication schedule. Authors were asked to include in their chapters, as applicable, the following considerations: ethics, standards, legal aspects, staffing issues and implications, differing practices as they apply to different types of libraries, research, evaluation, technology/automation, and budgeting and finance.

An extensive expert review process involved both academic and hospital librarians. Each volume includes a listing of the expert reviewers of that volume, in grateful acknowledgment of their efforts. The editor-in-chief and the editors are indebted to MLA's Managing Editor of Books, J. Michael Homan, for selecting reviewers and coordinating their work, and for his personal suggestions on organization, content, and format.

CPHSL is co-published by the Medical Library Association and Scarecrow Press, Inc. Special thanks are due to David B. Biesel, Director of Scarecrow's Association Publishing Program, Raymond S. Naegele, MLA's Director of Financial and Administrative Services, and Kimberly S. Pierceall, MLA's Director of Communications, for their advice and assistance. The indexing expertise of Beryl Glitz provides consistent and accurate access to the content of each volume.

Alison Bunting, Editor-in-Chief
Louise M. Darling Biomedical Library
University of California, Los Angeles

References

1. Doe J. ed. Handbook of medical library practice. Chicago: American Library Association, 1942:v.

2. Doe J, Marshall, ML, eds. Handbook of medical library practice. 2nd ed. Chicago: American Library Association, 1956.

3. Annan GL, Felter JW, eds. Handbook of medical library practice. 3rd ed. Chicago: Medical Library Association, 1970:v.

4. Ibid., vii.

5. Darling L, Bishop D, Colaianni LA, eds. Handbook of medical library practice. 4th ed. vol 1. Chicago: Medical Library Association, 1982: xi.

6. Ibid.

7. Ibid., xii.

8. Darling L, Bishop D, Colainni LA, eds. Handbook of medical library practice. 4th ed. vol. 3. Chicago: Medical Library Association, 1988: xiv.

9. Ibid.

10. Ibid., xv.

Expert Reviewers

Sandra L. Arnesen, Denver, CO
Jonathan D. Eldredge, Albuquerque, NM
Nancy B. Fazonne, Salem, MA
Frances H. Lynch, Nashville, TN
Jett McCann, Augusta, GA
Anne M. Pascarelli, Boston, MA
Lila Pedersen, Grand Forks, ND
Robert A. Pisciotta, Kansas City, KS
Cecile C. Quintal, Albuquerque, NM
Paula K. Turley, La Jolla, CA
Marjory A. Waite, Chapel Hill, NC

Advisory Committee Members

Rachael K. Anderson
Director, Health Sciences Center Library
University of Arizona
Tucson, AZ

Alison Bunting
Associate University Librarian for Sciences
Louise Darling Biomedical Library
University of California, Los Angeles
Los Angeles, CA

Dottie Eakin
Director, Medical Sciences Library
Texas A&M University
College Station, TX

Rick Forsman
Director, Denison Memorial Library
University of Colorado Health Sciences Center
Denver, CO

Ruth Holst
Director of Library Services
Medical Library
Columbia Hospital
Milwaukee, WI

J. Michael Homan
Director of Libraries
Mayo Foundation
Rochester, MN

Mary Horres
Associate University Librarian for Sciences
Biomedical Library
University of California, San Diego
La Jolla, CA

Kimberly Pierceall
Director of Communications
Medical Library Association
Chicago, IL

M. Sandra Wood
Librarian, Reference and Database Services
George T. Harrell Library
Milton S. Hershey Medical Center
Pennsylvania State University
Hershey, PA

Authors

Janis F. Brown
Associate Director, Educational Resources
Norris Medical Library
University of Southern California
Los Angeles, CA

Barbara A. Carlson
Head, Serials Management
Library
Medical University of South Carolina
Charleston, SC

Mark E. Funk
Head, Collection Development
Samuel J. Wood Library
Cornell University Medical College
New York, NY

Daniel H. Jones
Assistant Library Director for Collection Development
Briscoe Library
University of Texas Health Sciences Center at San Antonio
San Antonio, TX

David H. Morse
Associate Director, Collection Resources
Norris Medical Library
University of Southern California
Los Angeles, CA

Pat L. Walter
Associate Biomedical Librarian for Technical Services
Louise M. Darling Biomedical Library
University of California
Los Angeles, CA

Judith C. Wilkerson
Head of Serials Services
Robert M. Bird Health Sciences Center Library
University of Oklahoma
Oklahoma City, OK

Introduction

A book about health sciences library acquisitions practice in the 1990s faces some rather serious obstacles. For a start, the acquisition of books, serials, and media is arguably the most procedure-driven area of library operation and therefore the one in which library practice is most heterogeneous. It is also the area of library operation that partakes most of methods and disciplines borrowed from the broader arena of general business practice, and in which nearly all librarians are to some extent amateurs. Finally, it is the area of library practice that has been rendered most problematic by the advent of digital information sources that are made accessible to users but not actually "acquired" by the library.

For all of these reasons, the authors of the five chapters that constitute this volume have faced a uniquely difficult challenge in summarizing the state of "current practice" in biomedical libraries in a way that is both broadly applicable and yet specific enough to offer practical assistance. Adding to the difficulty of their task has been the need to take a Janus-like approach to the use of both manual and automated systems. The apparent reticence of acquisitions librarians in health science libraries to publish reports of their endeavors adds a final stumbling block to the would-be chronicler of current practice.

That the authors have succeeded as well as they have is a tribute to their many years of experience on the front line of acquisitions work and to their thorough understanding of the rapidly changing external forces that are and will be impacting the field in the years to come.

Viewed from the Olympian heights of information science theory, many of the issues presented in this volume may seen mundane, if not picayune. It is, however, the Editor's belief that it is on such undramatic matters as claiming cycles and bindery gluing methods that the library's ability to meet users' real needs often rests. For this reason, the chapter authors have been encouraged to emphasize practical how-to-do-it information and even prescriptive advice, rather than broad generalities and theoretical constructs.

Although the chapters are designed to stand as independent works, each in some way builds upon the chapters that precede it. Pat Walter's introductory chapter, for instance, treats those acquisition activities that are not specific to any single format of material, and it should therefore be read in conjunction with each of the format-specific chapters that follow. Similarly, Mark Funk's monograph acquisitions chapter introduces basic methods of ordering and receiving library materials that constitute the foundation for the discussion of serials and media acquisitions in the subsequent chapters.

Given the importance of serials in biomedical libraries, it seemed reasonable to devote two chapters to the subject. The chapter by Danny Jones and Judith Wilkerson focuses on the core serials acquisitions processes. Bobbie Carlson's chapter follows up with the post-acquisition serials procedures, such as bindery, missing issue replacement, and maintenance of holdings data. The final chapter on acquisition of audiovisual and machine-readable materials by Janis Brown and David Morse can be seen as an extension of all of the previous chapters into the era of the digital library.

If there is a predominant theme in these chapters it is that the acquisitions operation in health sciences libraries is only as good as the relationships it establishes — relationships with other departments of the library and the parent institution, with its automated system providers, with its books and serials vendors, with publishers, and with other libraries. The task of the acquisitions librarian is to understand and coordinate the resources of all of these groups toward the goal of eliminating barriers to information access.

Acknowledgments

The editor is deeply grateful to all of the chapter authors for their excellent work, their perseverance, and their unfailing good will throughout the long editorial review process; to the expert reviewers for their many helpful suggestions; and to Alison Bunting for her counsel and support.

1

Acquisitions—An Overview

Pat L. Walter

For users and most library staff, the acquisition of books, journals, CD-ROMs and other library materials is an obscure activity unfolding in a back room. The set of ordering and receiving functions that convert the intellectual choices of collection development into physical objects to be organized by catalogers is little understood and largely unremarked, especially if all runs well. But such a superficial view masks the underlying importance of the acquisitions process to library services, many of which will stand or fall depending on the quality and efficiency of acquisitions operations.

The basic acquisitions processes of gathering materials through buying, leasing, and even artful begging, pose complex and varied challenges. Whether in the large university library or the one-person hospital library, acquisitions staff contend with a multiplicity of sometimes obscure publishing sources, conducting business in a variety of fluctuating currencies. They deal with tax laws and licensure issues, with discounts and contracts; they must also satisfy institutional accountants and purchasing officers. The same staff is concerned with bibliographic verification and rules of entry, with the complexities of serials holdings statements and sequential titles, and with efficient utilization of national bibliographic utilities. Because the process-oriented tasks of acquisitions are prime targets for automation, efficient use of computer systems is added to the acquisition librarian's concerns.

It is the multifaceted nature of the acquisitions process that this chapter attempts to address. The aim is to define what is meant by acquisitions, what in general terms acquisitions functions entail, and how they fit into the library and the institutional structure. The chapter provides an introduction to the overall goals and strategies of acquisitions that underlie the format-specific expositions to follow in this volume. Additionally, the chapter addresses some of the external changes driving future expansions of acquisitions activities in libraries.

The Nature of Acquisitions

Defining Acquisitions

The acquisitions process has traditionally included those library functions that involve ordering, receiving, and paying for information materials that are to be added to the library's collection. These functions also include verifying that the desired materials actually exist, that the correct materials have been received, and that the appropriate funds are used to pay for them.

These traditional operations still constitute most of what acquisitions departments do, but the definition and concept of acquisition functions and processes are broadening [1-2]. In 1983 the Kronick and Bowden chapter in the 4th edition of the *Handbook of Medical Library Practice* concerned itself solely with acquiring materials for library ownership, and the materials they discussed were restricted to print, microforms, and audiovisuals [3]. Today, information materials needed for the biomedical library include printed or online books, subscriptions to print or electronic journals, CD-ROM products, and online databases of journal-article citations; other formats will certainly be added in the future. Moreover, materials need no longer reside in the library's collection to meet users' information needs. They may be stored remotely in digital form and be made available to patrons on demand, thereby making access to some information sources as important as their outright ownership.

A new, more inclusive, definition of acquisitions is emerging to embrace all library activities involved in the purchase, leasing, or otherwise obtaining legal access to information sources. Such a definition has the advantage of emphasizing the important common elements in activities such as book ordering, document delivery, or negotiating for access to a remote database; it may also provide the basis for a more efficient deployment of library personnel. Although the basic functions of verification, ordering, receiving, and paying have not changed, they may be exercised in more varied venues and for more varied types of information materials.

Having described what acquisitions is, it may be equally helpful to emphasize what it is not. Despite frequent blurring in the published literature and everyday use, acquisitions functions need to be differentiated from collection development. Acquisitions work does not concern itself with the selection of what should be acquired or made available to a library's clientele, nor with the decision on how funds should be expended, nor with the competing demands for collection dollars between journals and monographs, print and electronic media. All of these topics are discussed in the *Collection Development and Assessment in Health Sciences Libraries* volume of this series.

The inherent nature of integrated library automation systems contributes to blurring the distinctions between acquisitions and its closest functional neighbors, collection development and cataloging. The basic machine-readable record for an information item is often created in acquisitions, with at least preliminary decisions being made concerning access points and authority control, which are traditionally cataloging concerns. Similarly, decisions needing to be made by acquisitions personnel, such as how far to pursue the search for an elusive publication, require a solid understanding of the library's collection development priorities. The functions are intertwined, and in many cases so are the staff. In both large and small libraries, various steps of selecting, acquiring, and organizing material may be performed by the same people.

The essence of acquisitions lies in those functions that procure information for the use of library clientele and see to it that the information is appropriately paid for.

Professional Identity

A scan of the current literature reveals acquisitions librarians' uncertainty and soul-searching concerning their professional role—an introspection going well beyond general concern with the future of librarianship and the place of the library in an electronic world [4-6]. Acquisitions librarians feel buffeted in their role as intermediaries between collection development and the rest of the library, and between the library and the publishing world.

> ...acquisitions work, for a variety of reasons, tends to be undervalued and misunderstood; it may occupy a vulnerable position organizationally; it has minimal self-determination of its objectives and control of its work flow; and, regrettably, it receives less respect and exerts less influence than it deserves [7].

The undervaluation of acquisitions work stems from misperceptions and lack of familiarity. Library schools often ignore the field, focusing their restricted technical services emphasis on collection development and cataloging. And, unless acquisitions work is required as part of a "do everything" job, few librarians outside the acquisitions department are exposed to its many facets. Instead of appreciating the professional challenge of coordinating the bibliographic, automation, and business aspects of the acquisitions specialty, or of realizing the complexity of the book trade world in which the acquisitions librarian engages, the notion lingers in some quarters that the work is routine, process-oriented, and simple, requiring little more than supervision of clerks [8-9].

Although there is a fear that such attitudes may inhibit the future of acquisitions librarians in the evolving electronic library, there is no reason to think that such a development is inevitable. The fundamental role that the acquisition of materials plays in the traditional library holds true equally in a library without book stacks or print volumes, where the "materials" are "information," and where acquisitions may consist largely of arranging for access and contractual rights to such information. Meeting the challenges of the new digital era may indeed prove an opportunity to reestablish the acquisition function at the center of the library's mission. The scrutiny and self-searching the professional specialty is presently undergoing is a healthy sign of life. Acquisitions functions are being examined, as are all aspects of librarianship, in relation to new information resources and uses.

Learning and Keeping Up With Acquisitions

The practice of acquisitions is one of the less researched and documented aspects of library practice. Several helpful general monographs and edited collections have been published during the last few years, however, to aid the beginner and enlighten the experienced. In addition to the volumes focusing on acquisitions, some useful chapters are also available in works concerned with all of technical services.

Beginners can find basic information in the American Library Association's *Acquisition Guidelines* series started in 1973 [10] and still being published [11], and in the Miller how-to manual [12]. A more advanced treatment is provided by Magrill and Corbin in their comprehensive description of acquisitions management and collection development [13]. Among the more recent edited compilations, two deal substantively with evaluating acquisitions functions [14-15], while others discuss operational costs [16-17] and business aspects of acquisitions [18]. Katz's authors explore the role of, and relations with, vendors in the acquisitions process [19], while Genaway covers more general aspects of acquisitions [20]. The

Godden, Gorman, Leonhardt, and Racine compilations consider wider aspects of technical services [21-24]. Basch and Tuttle focus specifically on serials [25-26].

Much of the current serious thinking about the theory, practice, and future of acquisitions is first aired at some specific acquisitions/collection development conferences. Personal attendance at any of these gatherings is desirable, reading their proceedings is a must. The North American Serials Interest Group (NASIG) includes publishers, vendors, scholars, and librarians, all of whom are deeply concerned about the continuing health of scholarly publishing; meetings are held annually. The Charleston (South Carolina) Conference grew out of concern by librarians about the effects of steeply rising serials costs on the future of collections in large research libraries. Another annual gathering, the Feather River Institute sponsored by the University of the Pacific (California), focuses more specifically on the practice of acquisitions. The very active ALA special interest group, Association for Library Collections and Technical Services (ALCTS), sponsors a variety of specialized discussion groups at ALA meetings. Advance announcements and summaries, and often the entire proceedings, can be found in one or more of the journals cited below. The papers presented at these conferences pose the important questions of the acquisitions specialty, and the discussions they engender point the way to action.

Valuable print serials aimed at acquisitions librarians include *Library Acquisitions: Practice and Theory, The Acquisitions Librarian, The Serials Librarian, Serials Review,* and *Against the Grain.* (Issues of *The Acquisitions Librarian* are also packaged and promoted as monographs, requiring cautious ordering to avoid unwanted duplication.) The most efficient annual bibliography of acquisitions is provided in the third quarterly issue of *Library Resources and Technical Services;* and *The Bowker Annual of Library and Book Trade Information* provides a useful overview of trade happenings.

Electronic journals, newsletters, and bulletin boards are proliferating at such a rate that whatever information is provided here will quickly become outdated. However, these electronic exchanges, with their immediacy and interactive capability, are extremely useful, and some have become well established.

Health sciences acquisitions staff should become acquainted with the *Biomedical Library Acquisitions Bulletin* or *BLAB,* the electronic newsletter of the Medical Library Association's Collection Development Section [27]. A similar format is employed by *ACQNET,* an electronic newsletter aimed primarily at academic librarians [28]. The ALCTS's electronic newsletter, *ALCTS Network News* [29], supplements the printed ALCTS newsletter. One of the most influential of the electronic newsletters is Marcia Tuttle's *Newsletter on Serials Pricing Issues,* which goes well beyond pricing in its interests and which continues to be the venue for thoughtful commentaries and discussion [30]. Reading electronic mail and list servers devours time, but these are today's newspapers of the profession.

Acquisitions in the Health Sciences Library

The assignments of the librarian performing acquisitions functions in a health sciences library do not differ substantially from those performed in university or special libraries. A strong indicator of the similarity of acquisitions processes among libraries is the dearth of professional literature for specific types of libraries. The acquisitions literature is not large in any case, but even of that amount, only a tiny fraction is written by health sciences librarians or appears in health sciences journals. Under the *Bulletin of the Medical Library Association* index heading of "Acquisitions and Collection Development" almost no articles were listed during the years between 1983 and 1993 that pertained to acquisitions according to the definitions set in this chapter.

The acquisitions process is fundamentally the same in any library setting, irrespective of size of budget and staff or the type of clients served. Obtaining and paying for materials always anchors the process. Such differences as do emerge stem from the special characteristics of health sciences collections, on whether and what automated system is used, and other specifics of institutional operations. Which library department verifies requests before ordering, whether order records are visible to the public or not, whether the library is allowed to issue its own checks to pay vendors — each institution will provide a unique combination of answers to these and many other specific questions; but the answers will not differ substantially between health sciences and other types of libraries.

On the other hand, there are some distinctive aspects to health sciences library acquisitions. The ratio of money spent on books versus journals differs between the health sciences and other libraries; and nonprint formats may claim a greater role in the collection. The disciplines served by the health sciences library accord extraordinary importance to journal literature as a primary means of publication, and health sciences librarians recognize this distinction by maintaining subscriptions for major journals, whatever other materials they may have to forego. The extraordinarily high cost of medical books and journals burdens health sciences libraries and commands special care in every phase of the acquisitions process. Acquisitions personnel are aware that medical books have a limited lifespan, which puts a special premium on getting them to the shelves as soon as they are published; and gaps in the collection caused by inefficient or careless acquisitions procedures can have direct effects on patient care. This need to have the latest information available also makes the prompt claiming of missing journal issues not a luxury, but a rule of survival for the health sciences acquisitions staff.

Some health sciences libraries house great historical collections and actively continue to add to them. Others acquire only currently published scholarship in the history of medicine, and many bypass this area of collecting entirely. Consequently, the typical health sciences acquisitions librarian seldom needs the services of rare book dealers. Out-of-print dealers are also less often sought than in other types of libraries because of the general emphasis on providing current information and the prevalent pattern of publishing frequent new editions of medical texts.

Computer-aided instruction programs may demand much attention in the health sciences library, whereas some other special formats such as sound recordings are relatively rare. The mix of publishers from whom libraries purchase is also unique to the biomedical library, depending heavily on such exclusively biomedical houses as Saunders, Lippincott, and Williams & Wilkins. The prevalent use of vendors specializing in service to medical libraries is another distinguishing characteristic of the acquisitions process in biomedical libraries [31].

To summarize, although the process of acquiring materials in a health sciences library is not essentially different from that in other kinds of libraries, the types of materials acquired, and the specialized demands of the health sciences community, do give rise to some unique concerns and characteristic approaches.

The Context of Acquisitions

The acquisitions function plays a central role in the library in two senses. First, no library, especially no health sciences library, can exist without constantly replenishing its information store—which is the raison d'être for acquisitions. Secondly, acquisitions exists at the center of an overlapping and interconnecting universe of services and entities within and outside the parent institution. The quality of relationships between acquisitions and other library departments, and between acquisitions and the external world, are a good indicator of the quality of the acquisitions operation as a whole.

Acquisitions and the Biomedical Information Arena

The central acquisitions mission is to procure the materials that have been selected. To fulfill this mission effectively, it is useful for those involved in the process to have a basic understanding of the creation, production, and distribution of those materials—and of the symbiotic relationship that exists between those who produce and those who acquire biomedical information.

Primacy of the Biomedical Journal

The book may be the historian's or literary critic's primary tool, but for the biomedical researcher and physician the scientific journal article is the basic unit of information and of professional status. Faculty members' promotion and tenure decisions are based in large part on the number and quality of reports published in major refereed journals; publishing a book is a desirable adjunct, but not the precondition for career success it is for humanities or social sciences professors. Clinicians base their diagnosis and treatment on standards of practice as reflected in well-known and respected texts, but nevertheless are expected to keep up with current knowledge as published in major journals, and they may be liable to suit if they do not do so [32-33].

Beginning students in medicine, dentistry, and nursing formerly depended entirely upon their class syllabi and an armful of textbooks, but this is no longer the case. As problem-based learning increasingly dominates educational curricula, even first-year students are expected to consult journal articles for the latest information. Teaching how to evaluate the content of journal articles is one of the means of introducing and acclimating students to their profession. Graduate advisers organize journal clubs and tutorials to accomplish this, but in some locations librarians are now participating in, or even leading, this effort [34]. The primacy of the journal influences all aspects of health sciences library policies, from collection development to acquisitions to reference [35-37].

Users need tools to determine the content of this journal literature and they need to consult the articles themselves. As a gateway to journal content, the library provides access to indexing and abstracting tools, whether these be online, on CD-ROM or in print, on site or reached by telecommunication links. Of course the journals themselves must be acquired for the library or, to the degree that is not possible because of financial considerations, prompt delivery of specified articles must be made possible. Traditional interlibrary loan services, preferably speeded up by facsimile or other electronic transmission, may be used. These interlibrary transactions are increasingly being supplemented by use of commercial document delivery services.

The high cost of journals, and their continuing steep rate of price increase, are the major influences on acquisitions spending today and on the growth or nongrowth of the library collection. An enormous amount of effort has been devoted to analyzing this phenomenon [38-41]. Detailed knowledge of scientific serials, trends in their publishing and pricing, and familiarity with the publishers who produce them and the vendors who distribute them is an essential tool for the health sciences acquisitions librarian.

Biomedical Monographs and Other Media

From the primacy of journals in the health science setting arises the correlate that less money and time is expended on monographs. Any health sciences library needs a solid collection of standard texts in the medical disciplines, nursing, and other health fields that are represented within the institution. Such a basic collection demands augmentation and depth in those areas where residencies and other teaching programs are offered. In small hospital libraries the core volumes may be few indeed, but whatever the size of the book collection and the number of serials subscribed to, annual expenditures need to cover new editions to keep the standard works updated. Guaranteeing adherence to accepted standards of patient care, the first line of defense against malpractice suits, depends partially on following accepted expert opinion as documented in the current standard texts and peer-reviewed articles.

In larger collections other types of monographs and perhaps a few conference proceedings join the core textbooks. Specialized teaching materials such as outlines, study guides, and examination questions may be acquired. Government documents, especially statistics, regulations, and practice guidelines, are of special importance in the health sciences. Much of the world's scientific publication appears in English, whether published in the U.S., Europe, or elsewhere; thus buying non-English materials occupies only a minuscule role in the average health sciences acquisitions department.

The mix of publication formats in the health sciences library, other than the pervasively high journal-to-book ratio, depends upon the particular educational, research, and patient care responsibilities of the institution. Although print is still the most important medium, it is no longer the only one to collect. Microforms, audiovisuals, and CD-ROM are already found in the majority of health sciences libraries, and computer-aided instruction programs, electronic journals, videodiscs, and emerging technologies for information packaging will assume increasing importance.

The Role of Publishers and Vendors

The roles of publishers, vendors, and the acquisitions department in serving information creators and users are reasonably well defined [42], although the financial effects of these players' involvement on the ultimate costs of biomedical information are more controversial.

Researchers, clinicians, educators—a host of basic and clinical health sciences professionals create knowledge through their work. That knowledge is transcribed into information units to be passed on to others. At present, the usual course is to give those units to publishers who package the intellectual content and market the packages. Frequently, but not always, publishers enhance the intellectual content through editorial planning and revision. Publishers also search the scientific plains for uncultivated patches and enlist authors and editors to fill perceived gaps in coverage. Whether this results in useful dissemination of scientific thought or in unnecessary publication depends on the point of view of the commentator and evaluation of the specific work in question.

Health sciences libraries serve the professionals and students who are interested in the content of these information products, and therefore libraries need to buy them or gain access to them through some other means. To ease the labor of dealing with the existing multitude of publishers, most libraries utilize the services of vendors, who act as middlemen and facilitators between the worlds of publishers and libraries. Vendors add value to the products they handle—whether books, journals, or CD-ROM—by making them more convenient for libraries to obtain; it is much easier to be invoiced once for a consolidated list of journal subscriptions than to have to deal with individual orders and invoices from each publisher.

The interests of libraries and vendors overlap because both want libraries to prosper and keep buying materials. It would seem that publishers' interests, also, overlap with those of libraries, but questions have arisen whether publishers see it so. Some recent practices such as drastic price increases, extreme differentials in prices charged to libraries and to individuals, proliferation of duplicative titles, and the unchecked increase in number of pages published by established journals, might make one think otherwise. As the financial picture worsens, vendors can play an important role in controlling costs and as advocates for the library community [43-45].

The acquisitions librarian enters into a contract, written or implied, with the vendor on behalf of the library, through which the library expects to obtain prompt delivery of materials, for which it will be billed a reasonable price. Although contractual aspects of the library-vendor process differ somewhat from the sale of general goods, they are not so unique as to require a special legal code. The Uniform Commercial Code, supplemented by case law and the Restatement (Second) of 1981, covers vendor-library sales [46]. Business aspects of librarians as consumers are discussed by Marsh [47]. In many academic and hospital health sciences libraries, no specific written contract for services is signed; the purchase order sent to vendor or publisher for a list of materials serves as the equivalent.

The Library-Vendor Relationship

The authors of the succeeding chapters will describe in more detail the specifics of living with or without vendors—how to choose them and how to evaluate them. Here the purpose is only to introduce some general questions to consider: whether to use a vendor at all or to obtain materials directly from their producers; whether to use only one vendor or to divide business among several and, if several, which orders should go to whom? How does one judge vendor performance? Finally, the acquisitions librarian needs an understanding of how to optimize library-vendor relationships and what principles of business ethics apply.

What is it that a vendor really provides? A vendor can supply experience and know-how, efficiency, convenience, discounted prices, technological expertise, cost-effectiveness, automation options, communication links, training, and occasionally some clout with publishers; in bad times, a vendor might even extend credit at the end of the year. The serials vendor bundles tens or hundreds of separate subscription invoices into one; the monograph vendor provides titles from hundreds of different publishers.

Vendors offer many kinds of service. Libraries choose those that will maximize benefits in terms of financial and staff costs. For their services the vendor may or may not charge a service fee, and the equation will be beneficial to the library if the sum of savings in staff time and discounts earned is more than the sum of the service fee [48]. For monographs, libraries want the service that can provide the largest proportion of the books needed for the library's clientele [49]. Librarians not only demand efficient and accurate service, but also expect technological sophistication, and access to automated systems [50], such as electronic interfaces to automated library systems, vendor-designed serials check-in systems, or databases of publishing information on books and journals. Additional services available from vendors are periodic spending summaries and analyses of materials bought, notifications of new publications, budget projections, and claiming of unreceived serials issues or books from publishers.

Libraries "…value vendors for their attention to detail, tenacity, precision, efficiency, friendliness, and scope of service as well as their speed and overall effectiveness in obtaining the books" [51]. "A successful library-vendor relationship has to be based on shared priorities and goals that define specified services to the library and frequent, honest, and effective communication between the organizations' representatives" [52].

Whether to buy directly from publishers or to use one or several vendors must be based strictly on local conditions, guided mainly by the size of the acquisitions effort and the heterogeneity of the materials acquired. Even a small library can gain from using vendor services, but a small hospital library might find it an undue complication to deal with more than one vendor for the number of books and subscriptions it orders.

The solution is less obvious for the large academic library with a million-dollar acquisitions budget. The parameters for purchasing decisions set down by the institution's purchasing department may channel or even dictate the decision. In some institutions, one may choose only from a list of approved suppliers; in others, all purchases must be bid on, and the nod goes to the lowest bidder. Government libraries, especially those in the federal government, usually are constrained with very explicit and strict parameters for purchasing.

If organizational rules do not point the way, prudence, common sense, and careful investigation must be the guide. The library wants the best deal possible: can a single vendor provide all the subjects needed by the library? All the formats? Does the vendor with the desired serials check-in system also supply books? Does only one vendor's automated system feed smoothly into the library's system? Is the discount on overseas books better from an overseas vendor? Does one vendor accept payment in dollars whereas another will not? Will dividing the orders according to various vendors' specialties result in an overall saving?

Most large libraries find themselves dealing with more than one vendor, at the least splitting their business between serials and monograph special-ists. Some firms that deal exclusively in health sciences materials have given excellent service to many health sciences libraries who need, even so, to turn to additional dealers for materials outside this subject area.

If the vendors' role is to provide service, they must be judged upon the quality and quantity of such service. Criteria to be considered include cost effectiveness, convenience, speed of service, specialized expertise, and the fit of subjects and formats provided to the needs of the collection. The information gathered in a study of vendor performance, both comparisons of one firm against another and a closer analysis of a single firm over an extended period of time, has value for the library beyond the obvious; as with any close look at library operations, it can provide enlightening insights into procedures and open the way for improvements [53].

The literature of library-vendor relations is fairly extensive [54-56]. All of the major texts on library acquisitions include at least one chapter on library-vendor interaction, and the largest cluster of acquisitions-related journal articles focuses on this topic. Fisher provides a brief history of the last forty years of library-vendor relations, and has some pungent com-ments about current conditions and hindrances to the relationship [57]. Looking into the future, some authors see new and much expanded roles for vendors, such as contracting with the library to assume all acquisitions functions [58].

Ethics in the Library-Vendor Relationship

As shrinking library budgets call forth extraordinary ingenuity to make them stretch, and vendors battle for business to stay alive, the ethical relationship between librarian and vendor is an old topic gaining new importance. Acquisitions work has been characterized as "people with no money [the acquisitions librarian] interacting with people trying to make money [the vendor]" [59], a situation that naturally creates conditions where suspicions may arise. Ethical behavior should be built upon the fundamental characteristics of honesty, professional integrity, good business practice, and respect for people and organizations [60]. One writer advises librarians not to get into "situations in which personal interests might be served or financial benefits gained at the expense of library users, colleagues, or the employing institutions." Yet, even as librarians are warned to keep their distance, he goes on to say, they continuously approach vendors for various forms of financial support, such as scholarships, awards, prizes, and sponsorship of professional meetings [61].

The questions on an ethics survey administered to librarians and vendors provide a neat summary of potentially troublesome areas in library-vendor relations:

1. Do social events obligate a library or acquisitions librarian?
2. Is it fair to compare your vendor contracts with those of other libraries?
3. What information should vendors reveal among themselves about libraries?
4. What information should vendors reveal to libraries about other vendors?
5. What are legitimate promises on both sides? [62].

Question number four above could be expanded to add "...or about other libraries?", although this particular area of confidentiality is thorny. Who does not enjoy talking about mutual acquaintances and what is happening in one's own and other institutions? And when does that talk cross the line to betrayal of confidential information?

Accepting the hospitality of vendors at a meal or in their convention hotel suite is common among librarians, and therefore its ethical dimension is also a common topic of debate. An open discussion of this question by librarians and vendors has elicited responses ranging all the way from "I never accept anything so there can never be a question" to "I don't think an occasional meal is going to corrupt me." The most common view seems to be that the exercise of common sense and a professional attitude will maintain ethical standards [63]. Various other topics one may not immediately connect with ethics are covered by chapters in the Strauch compilation [64-65].

This question of appropriate business ethics for acquisitions librarians has been of major concern to the ALCTS Acquisitions Section, which has drafted a statement on Principles and Standards of Acquisitions Practice which was discussed at the 1993 ALA conference. The text of the draft statement follows:

An acquisitions librarian:

1. Gives first consideration to the objectives and policies of his or her library.
2. Strives to obtain the maximum ultimate value of dollar of expenditure.
3. Grants all competing vendors equal consideration insofar as the established policies of his or her library permit, and regards each transaction on its own merits.
4. Subscribes to and works for honesty, truth, and fairness in buying and selling, and denounces all forms and manifestations of commercial bribery.
5. Uses only by consent original ideas and designs devised by one vendor for competitive purchasing purposes.
6. Accords a prompt and courteous reception insofar as conditions permit to all who call on legitimate business missions.
7. Fosters and promotes fair, ethical and legal trade practices.
8. Strives consistently for knowledge of the publishing and bookselling industry.
9. Strives to establish practical and efficient methods for the conduct of his or her office.
10. Counsels and assists fellow acquisitions librarians in the performance of their duties, whenever occasion permits [66].

Acquisitions Within the Library Organization

Organizational Alignments

Where in the library organizational structure does the acquisitions operation fit? With what other similar functions should it be allied? To whom should its head report? The literature provides many different descriptions which may show trends, but provide no overall definitive answers [67-74].

The reason, of course, is that the answers depend upon the type of institution, the size of the library, the space configuration, the automated system, and the acquisitions budget. A separate acquisitions department, division, or section may not be the right solution for a specific library—in smaller libraries acquisitions functions may constitute only a part of one individual's overall job. If there is a separate section, its traditional placement has been squarely within the technical services division, alongside cataloging; collection development may or may not make it a triad.

The main goal for the internal organization of technical services is to maximize functional interactions. Selection, acquisition, and bibliographic organization all center on the bibliographic record, supplying a reason for grouping these functions together [75-76]. Familiarity with and use of the same record also facilitate cross-training of staff in a number of tasks. Such cross-training provides variety and widens understanding of what is being done and why; the outcome is enhanced efficiency of the whole [77]. Pre-order searching can easily be integrated with collection development procedures, and collection development staff could perform both functions. Similarly, determining form of entry and authoritative form of names and series easily fits into the record-entry phase of acquisitions, but these are also traditional cataloging tasks frequently assumed by that department.

Opinion on whether serials and monograph acquisitions should be combined or separate is not uniform, but unification seems to be right for some libraries [78]; there are also suggestions for consolidating all acquisitions functions, regardless of format, source, cost, or eventual location of materials [79]. One study has surveyed technical services organization in sixteen libraries, in many of which technology encouraged the merging of monographic and serials acquisitions. An additional finding of the study was that the lines between acquisitions and cataloging seemed to be blurring, but collection development was generally still considered as a discrete function [80-81].

A variety of other realignments of technical services have been reported. Some authors describe a closer relationship between acquisitions and collection development, with acquisitions reporting to the head of collection development [82]. Another model involves the merging of collection development and acquisitions and the dissolution of a separate serials section [83]. In one institution, reorganization along subject lines distributed cataloging to each of the library's three subject divisions, but centralized acquisitions by moving serials maintenance into it. Experimentation with cataloging upon receipt in the acquisitions section may add even more functions in the future [84-85].

Outside pressures—changing technology, new types of information with new uses, tighter budgets and the resultant need for leaner organizations—will continue to dictate a reexamination of all the traditional alignments. An emerging trend is to eschew the dichotomy between public and technical services; new groupings may pair user services with collection services, or information access with information organization. Certainly no new standard of library organization has yet emerged, but some acquisitions departments may expect to find themselves with new and strange bedfellows in the future. Consideration of such realignments and their benefit-cost ratio are as important for the small as for as the large library.

Interdepartmental Relationships

In addition to the obvious ties to collection development and cataloging, acquisitions is also linked surprisingly strongly with public services departments. The reference staff are frequent and demanding users of acquisitions information—on-order records and serial check-in records, for example—because they face user questions regarding the availability of library materials. Special collections and nonprint materials divisions sometimes select and even order their own materials from specialty dealers, but equally often depend on the acquisitions division to receive and pay for those materials.

With interlibrary loan and document delivery departments the relationship may be a financial one, in which acquisitions pays interlibrary borrowing bills along with other invoices. Or it may evolve into a much more elaborate symbiosis based on the principle that both acquisitions and book or article delivery from outside sources procure information for users and thus their functions can and perhaps should be merged [86].

A close and dependent connection exists between acquisitions and a library's systems department, programmer, or automation guru [87]. The clerical, sequential, and monetary aspects of acquisition functions lend themselves particularly well to automation; especially in locally designed integrated library systems, the processing modules were the first to be designed [88]. As automated library systems evolve and networking becomes more widespread, technological developments centered on direct electronic data interchange among vendors, acquisitions, and accounting departments will only increase the need for such strong ties.

Total quality management may or may not be the current ruling passion in a particular institution, but a high level of quality control is mandatory for running a good organization. That control must, of course, be exercised at all levels and in all quarters of the library, but it is particularly critical in acquisitions, just because so many different groups use and depend on acquisitions information. With everyone online to the integrated library system, steps of the acquisitions process can be tracked and timed precisely by all with access to the system. Easily visible inefficiencies and inaccuracies can quickly sour relationships with colleagues and patrons.

To obtain the exact monograph requested by a selector and not some similar-sounding text by another author; to assure that occasional supplements to a journal are actually received and linked with the correct publication; to make sure that information passed to cataloging is complete and accurate; to make reserve materials available when the teaching semester starts—these are some of the imperatives in sustaining the acquisitions department's credibility within the library. To fulfill them, the person responsible for acquisitions operations must ensure that records are kept meticulously, that staff understand and follow procedures, and that no backlogs develop or problem situations lie hidden in file drawers. Quality control in acquisitions demands follow-up —systematic claiming and double-checking by the automation system whenever possible, manual "tickler" files, and comprehensive record review when needed. Promptness, accuracy and thoroughness are the qualities that will foster mutually productive relationships with other library departments.

Acquisitions and the Parent Institution

Acquisitions has been characterized as the hub within the library wheel and the bridge reaching out to the commercial world of information production and distribution. In addition, there are entities within the parent institution to which the acquisitions department connects more closely than do other departments of the library. These entities are the business offices of purchasing and accounting; the organization's computing facility; and in an academic setting, the student book store. Acquisitions staff may also need to contact other experts in the institution on specific occasions. One example is the legal department, which may be required to review licensing agreements to assure that they do not conflict with institutional rules.

Purchasing Departments

Libraries are rarely in a position to conduct financial transactions directly with their suppliers, such as publishers or vendors. Usually they must work through the parent institution's purchasing and payment bureaucracy. Unfortunately, relations with institutional business offices can sometimes be sources of complication and delay. Maintaining smooth relations between the library and its business office partners demands understanding of each other's ways and, on the library's part, an understanding of the institution's rules of doing business and a willingness to follow them.

These rules may seem excessively complex or even counterproductive, because purchasing 100 books is not the same as purchasing 100 cartons of paper or contracting for 100 hours of painting. Most of an institution's business is of this latter kind, however, and the librarian may need to seek a face-to-face meeting with a purchasing officer to explain the library's special circumstances and needs. The desired outcome of such a consultation is, at the least, to be allowed to order from publishers, vendors, or book stores directly and to be able to issue official purchase orders that do not require prior approval by the purchasing office. It may also be beneficial to seek authority for making payment directly to the supplier without going through the financial department.

It is equally or even more vital to win the right not to go through a periodic bidding process because a year's total purchase of books or journals exceeds some preset dollar figure. Changing the serials vendor each year because of a new low bid constitutes an acquisition librarian's nightmare. Nor does the library want to be forced to break purchases into separate small units so as not to exceed a single-purchase ceiling imposed by the institution. Even without such extreme constraints, many institutions demand a renewal of "blanket" requisitions at the beginning of each year for major vendors. Federal and local government hospital libraries suffer particularly from restrictive rules governing purchasing. If the rules have been made locally, a vigorous attempt to educate the decision makers is certainly called for. If the rules have been made by administrators far away, at several levels removed from the individual library, the battle may not be worth undertaking.

Accounting Departments

An understanding reached with the purchasing department at least endures for a considerable time, until the education process must be renewed with a new purchasing officer. However, talk may do little to solve problems with the accounting department if, through lack of luck or planning, the institution's accounts payable practices do not mesh with the library's operational needs or, even worse, with its automated system.

The library needs to pay its suppliers as quickly as possible, because meeting standard invoice deadlines may earn a discount; if it is impossible to meet the thirty- or sixty-day terms, discounts may be lost or finance charges added. Unfortunately, when unhappy suppliers complain about not having been paid—and for small publishers this can cause real hardship—they seldom call the accounting department. They call the library acquisitions department staff, who find it difficult to explain that they have done all within their power to speed the payment on its way and that the matter is now in someone else's hands.

The problem may lie with the size and practices of the institution, which interject delays of excessive verification between approval of payment and sending a check, or insufficient accounts payable staff may be unable to keep up with the workload. The delays may arise from automated systems which are unable to communicate with each other, requiring repeated input of the invoice information—first into the library's fund accounting system and then again into the accounting department's system. Could the computers communicate, and were they permitted to communicate when they technically can, numbers could flow from one system to the next, and the check would really be in the mail on time.

The literature carries both horror and success stories of library-accounting office interactions in an automated environment [89-90]. One of the unhappy stories concerns a library and accounting office whose systems did not interface well, and internal politics prevented a programming solution to the incompatibility. But from the experience the author distilled excellent advice on how to plan for a successful interaction:

- Involve the institution's internal auditors before buying or designing the library's automated system.

- Don't compromise. Insist on a system that will be useful for the library. The library is not a service agency for the accounting department; it's the other way around.

- Librarians know more about automation than do accountants. Hold out for a truly efficient linkage between systems.

- Keep a vision before you, of "a completely paperless payment process: no paper invoices, no paper ledgers, and no paper checks" [91].

It is clear that data consistency is imperative for a successful interface between automated systems. Different data elements may be needed by the two systems, but the common elements should exist in a consistent format in each system. As an example, the code in the library system that indicates from whom the material was acquired should match the code in the accounting system which indicates to whom payment should be sent [92].

Managing prompt payment for materials is not the only accounting practice with which the acquisitions librarian needs familiarity. There is also the audit trail—"a documentary history of an authorized order" [93]. A "documentary history" allows for step-by-step reconstruction of all financial decisions for each collection item ordered by the library. An "authorized order" demands the name or initials of the person, usually the collection development librarian, who requested the item's ordering. Other steps in the acquisitions process which may require documented authorization are allocation and transfer of funds, and invoice approval. Auditors are also concerned that only authorized staff have the power to alter data in financial fields of the record.

An institution may require that such documentary history exist on paper, although such a requirement is fast disappearing; the usual practice now is to accept as sufficient the financial information recorded on the item's machine-readable record in the library system. This practice of course has implications for format and accessibility of the record—demanding not only that specific fields be available for audit-related information, but that records be maintained for as long as the institution's accounting practices require.

Accounting standards are established for both private- and public-sector organizations in the U.S. by the Financial Accounting Standards Board (FASB). The American Institute of Certified Public Accountants (AICPA) issues guidelines which may be useful to librarians needing to design an accounting system [94].

A clear and thorough explanation of audit demands and the stresses and opportunities they afford between the library and institutional accounting officers is presented by Hawks. After an exposition of the internal controls available and the issues and procedures involved in auditing an automated acquisitions system, Hawks concludes

> Controls over access to data fields and equipment play a larger role in the audit process than most libraries would expect. The ability to control access to data files and to control enhancements to the software by the vendor is a critical area of concern for an auditor [95].

Applicable control mechanisms for keeping data safe may include segregating various functions and using different passwords to access each function; requiring authorization for transactions; and maintaining a log of all record updating activities. Rigorous administration of password security is a prerequisite.

Just as library staff make occasional errors in posting invoices and linking payment to specific book funds, so do institutional accounting staff, and libraries may want a way to double-check the accuracy of institutional financial reports. In most cases libraries protect themselves by running their own fund accounting system—usually through the automated acquisitions system, but occasionally by manual ledger entries. Such an internal accounting system should also allow instant determination of book fund balances. These balances may not match exactly those reported by the accounting department, because of the time lag between authorizing payment and the actual issuing of the check, but they should be a close approximation of fund status. Such an easily accessible internal system becomes a life-saver as the end of the payment year approaches and the size of remaining balances becomes critical.

Computing Facilities

Whether a library's acquisitions unit deals directly with the institution's computing staff depends entirely upon the local organization of computing resources. Some libraries have their own systems and programming staff who take care of library needs and handle necessary communications with outside computer and network groups. In other cases, each library division deals directly with a campus computing entity. It may be helpful, therefore, to summarize the demands that acquisitions, by the nature of its work, makes beyond the bounds of the library's integrated automated system.

The major demands are for interconnectivity and interfacing with outside computer systems—be they in the accounting department or in the vendors' or publishers' warehouses. Since acquisitions deals in commercial transactions, it needs convenient access to the commercial world's systems. The preferable connectivity is a fully automated one of computer-to-computer electronic data interchange (EDI). But until electronic data interchange according to universally accepted standards becomes an everyday reality, the immediate need may be for programming of interfaces between systems, mapping and translating data from one system to feed automatically into the other system. It is incumbent on acquisitions staff to be alert for opportunities to speed and simplify their work by technological means. They should work with the computing staff and outside entities such as vendors to draw up specifications for useful automation enhancements.

Campus Book Stores

A book store to supply titles for the individual needs of the institution's population is often found on a university or separate medical campus. Its inventory can be of great help to the acquisitions operation in the health sciences library, and a close relationship with the store's manager should be cultivated. When a professor's reserve reading list comes in one day before the start of classes, or the *Physician's Desk Reference* and *Merck Manual* are stolen from the reference desk, the usual procurement processes may be too slow to satisfy user demand. The convenience of walking to the book store and picking up the replacement volume with nothing but an interdepartmental purchase order in hand is invaluable. This is possible if a previous agreement about allowable purchasing shortcuts has been reached between parties.

It is frequently claimed that publishers and vendors favor the lucrative book store business over that of libraries, and ship new titles first to their commercial customers. True or not, it does seem that the campus book store sometimes has new medical titles or editions in hand before the library sees them. An understanding with the store's management can reserve copies for the library and thus save the library from the embarrassment of being without titles prominently displayed in the campus store. The speed and ease of dealing with the book store arises from it being essentially a retail transaction; that usually means there is little or no discount from the retail price. Cost versus expediency must be balanced in deciding when book store purchases may be an advantage.

If hospitals have a book store, its usual aim is to serve patients and visitors; rarely would it stock material of interest to the hospital library. But it might behoove that library to cultivate relations with a technical book store nearby, for the same reasons the academic library would—the need to pick up an occasional volume very quickly and without red tape.

Acquisitions and Other Institutions

Cooperative Agreements

Most interinstitutional library agreements are forged to serve areas other than acquisitions—cooperative collection development, reciprocal access and borrowing privileges, reference referrals, or cooperative interlibrary loan and document delivery agreements. However, cooperative agreements, both formal and informal, do have an impact on acquisitions operations.

Cooperative buying of books and journals is one area where an acquisitions unit can usefully join with its counterparts in similar institutions to gain advantages of size. Several nearby libraries can form consortia to negotiate price breaks for volume purchases by contracting with the same vendor, either submitting one joint approval profile for their combined needs or individual profiles. The increased number of titles acquired, perhaps in multiple copies, allows negotiation of a better discount than any one library would receive separately. The advantage can be heightened if a central receiving point is designated, thus making shipping easier and cheaper for the vendor. Before entering into such an agreement the library should weigh its advantages against such potential negatives as extra record keeping, time lost in negotiations, and potential loss of control and spontaneity.

Cooperative buying agreements make sense for small libraries banding together to gain strength, but they may be equally advantageous for large libraries. Especially when dealing with large database or CD-ROM producers, for example, cooperative purchase of multiple copies and cooperative access agreements that cover several libraries on one or on separate campuses can augment buying power.

Shared collection development among institutions can be organized along subject lines, by publisher, by countries of publication, by type of publication, or any other logical division—from the point of view of the acquisitions operation the particular specialization assigned its library does not matter very much. Whatever it may be, extra expertise in procuring the materials of that specialty must be developed. For complete subject coverage, the publishers and vendors, societies and associations, and out-of-print journal dealers specializing in that subject need to be identified and cultivated. If the assigned specialty is a publisher or a country, specific contacts must be made to acquire materials consistently and expeditiously.

Cooperative collecting should not alter greatly the number of items the acquisitions staff needs to process, because spreading the load evenly among participating institutions is a usual goal of such agreements. But participating in any cooperative approach entails extra work because of the added reporting and record keeping involved. Someone in the cooperative will be collecting information on number, cost, and ownership of titles acquired, in order to assure financial equity [96].

Similar responsibilities to report information on a periodic schedule result from membership in a union list of serials holdings. Additions and deletions of titles, usually including specific holdings, are supplied to a central agency in a specified format. Or, again as a facet of cooperative collection development, advance notice may be sent to a central listing of new serial titles the library is intending to buy or to cancel. The acquisitions department rarely negotiates such agreements, but frequently is expected to assume the obligations of documentation and reporting [97].

Programs for exchange of duplicate journal issues are a form of cooperation directly serving acquisitions functions. Whether organized by a professional society such as the Medical Library Association or one of its regional chapters, or a nonprofit organization like the United States Book Exchange, or set up as a commercial service like The Faxon Company's SerialsQuest, a serials exchange depends upon the willingness of its members or customers to list unwanted serials issues and to order wanted ones. The work of organization, data input, and record maintenance that acquisitions personnel freely contribute make serials exchanges a good source for inexpensive replacement issues and volumes.

Professional Organizations

In addition to the advantages that may accrue from participation in cooperative duplicate exchange programs sponsored by professional associations, involvement in professional organizations can bring wider benefits to the institution as well as the individual. Cooperative and collective action can be promoted through such groups as the Publishing and Information Industries Relations Committee (PIIRC) of the Medical Library Association, the MLA's Technical Services or Collection Development

Sections, the relevant bodies of the American Library Association, and the National Information Standards Organization (NISO). These bodies can address acquisition librarians' concerns about publisher and vendor practices, pricing, and promulgation of standards more effectively than can any single library.

Acquisitions and the User

Connections between the acquisitions staff and the user are mostly indirect—usually by way of collection development or reference intermediaries—except when acquisitions staff are asked to notify users directly when a desired book or journal issue is received. In some institutions, however, the library takes on the task of ordering books and serials for any individual or department within the institution, regardless of whether the expenditure is charged to the library budget; in such cases, of course, the acquisitions department will see and hear more directly from its extra-library constituencies. Even without such an official assignment, the acquisitions unit may expect occasional seekers of advice on purchasing or leasing materials, since it is perceived as the focus of commercial expertise in the library.

Some libraries are experimenting with staffing public information desks with personnel from units other than reference, including acquisitions staff. This staff's familiarity with searching the online catalog and ability to interpret automated records makes acquisitions personnel valuable resources in such assignments. The staff also often welcomes the public contact, which broadens their experience and frame of reference.

Acquisitions departments also may be the producers of certain lists or databases that are made available to the library user, such as lists of items at the bindery or in other stages of processing, or new book lists. In designing such tools, staff should be responsive to the needs of library users.

The real challenge for acquisitions supervisors is not in dealing with the occasional face-to-face public interaction, but in fostering a departmental spirit that keeps the needs of the library user constantly in mind. Acquisitions staff should never forget whom they serve—not themselves and not the rest of the library staff, but the library user.

The Basic Elements of Acquisitions

The basic tasks of the acquisitions process have become reasonably standardized in biomedical libraries. Because later chapters will address the specifics of this process, it will suffice here to name and briefly define the multiple facets of traditional acquisitions work. A discussion of future extensions and evolutions of such work will follow.

Bibliographic Functions

Some authors ponder whether the bibliographic aspects of acquisitions work are losing importance, since so much good bibliographic information is provided by national utilities, publishers, or vendors. They believe that what truly distinguishes acquisitions librarians and defines their specialty is their business skills [98]. The usual job description for an acquisitions head, however, still balances business and bibliography in fairly equal terms.

Preorder Searching

The term "preorder searching" includes two goals, which may be carried out at different times and by different staffs depending on the work flow and organization of the specific institution.

The first goal is to obtain a reliable and complete bibliographic description of the desired item; most publishers' catalogs and vendor lists, as well as some published reviews, may suffice to provide this. But badly garbled or erroneous requests do come to acquisitions for purchase—a half-complete, half-legible note, a passing reference in a news story, or any one of the hundred other ways partial information becomes the only available starting point. Then some inspired detective work becomes necessary, drawing on national bibliographic utilities, printed sources of all kinds, phone calls to the original requestor and to possible publishers—whatever is necessary to provide further clues. However, guidelines to limit the time spent on a bad reference are needed as a practical safeguard.

The second goal of preorder searching establishes that the desired item is not already held in the collection. Several access points for each publication should be searched in the library's online or card catalog, including author, title, and series title. Given the high cost of library materials, it pays to invest an extra few minutes of staff time to avoid a costly duplicate. At this stage the checker may also record the presence in the collection of related works, such as previous editions.

Creating the Order Record

As soon as an item has been ordered, or as an integral part of the ordering process, a record is created. Order slips can be typed on multiple-copy forms and filed into an in-process file; but in present-day libraries the in-process file is usually online in one of the myriad micro-, mini-, or mainframe automated systems in existence. The user and the rest of the library staff can have notice of the material's order as soon as it has been placed.

The order record can trigger a printed or electronically transmitted purchase order, and its presence in the on-order file should prevent future duplicate orders. In an automated system it also frequently serves a more important and lasting function—it becomes the basis for the final cataloged record. This characteristic of integrated library systems, that a record once created is progressively transformed to serve different functions, has profound impact on the importance of the acquisitions process. If the order record will soon be the cataloged record, it seems only efficient and cost effective to create the best possible record from the beginning. Thus, familiarity with MARC tagging, name authority, and rules of entry have became necessary for acquisition personnel, giving them a new level of responsibility and visibility.

Business Functions

Acquisition By Purchase

Purchasing books, journals, and media is still the most common way of acquiring them, and this function can be performed in a variety of ways. The library may use approval plans, blanket orders, and firm orders or, most commonly, a combination of these. Because these methods of buying also function as methods of selecting what to buy, collection development and acquisitions staff must cooperate in choosing the most efficacious approach.

In an approval plan, the vendor selects and supplies materials according to the library's profile of interest. The profile may set limits by subject matter, country of publication, publisher, cost, level of material, format, or any combination thereof. The agreement can specify that certain materials be sent sight unseen while for others a printed description on a standardized form should be submitted first for the library's decision; this latter method is sometimes called a "slips service." It is agreed that the library has the right to return materials that it feels do not meet its profile or are unwanted for other reasons, but an approval plan is not really successful for either library or vendor if too high a percentage of returns occurs [99]. Serials are normally excluded from approval plans, except for first volumes of new numbered series.

A blanket order is more general than an approval plan, usually covering all publications within broad subject areas and specified formats from a country or geographic region. One type of blanket order focuses on all publications of one publisher, usually a professional society or governmental body. Unlike an approval plan, a blanket order usually does not permit return of unwanted items.

Both the approval plan and the blanket order leave the actual choice of titles to the vendor or publisher, within the parameters set by the library. The library is spared the considerable labor cost of having to select each individual title it wants to purchase, and it achieves wider coverage than it could hope to attain on its own. In addition, approval plan vendors offer discounts on most publishers' titles.

A firm order is what it sounds like—a specific order for a specific title, sent to publisher, agent, or vendor. Firm ordering is the most common method for ordering serials, media formats, and, in smaller libraries, for books. It is also the slowest, most labor-intensive, and therefore costly, method of purchase. However, the availability of online ordering services through book vendors is transforming this method to a more viable option even for larger libraries.

Acquisition By Other Means

Aside from purchase, materials may also be acquired by deposit, gift, exchange, or through a licensing agreement.

Acquisition By Deposit

Depository arrangements with the U. S. Government Printing Office (GPO) assure that all GPO-distributed government documents in series or groups previously selected by the depository library arrive automatically and free of charge. In return, the library is responsible for providing free access to such documents to the public, irrespective of other access restrictions it may enforce. Strict retention obligations for all deposit materials exist and acquisitions staff must be meticulous in conforming to such retention rules. Health sciences libraries will have no interest in being a full depository for the entire range of government documents. The ideal arrangement, either in concert with a university's main depository library or negotiated directly, is to become a partial depository for health-related materials. Similar arrangements for state government documents may also be available.

It must be noted that the U.S. government is rethinking its entire information program with the dual goals of achieving better information distribution and cutting costs [100-101]. Certainly many more materials will be distributed in electronic and microform formats in the future. What role commercial companies will play in packaging and distribution of government information is a topic being hotly debated [102-103].

Acquisition By Donation

The ambiguous blessing of journal and book gifts come to all libraries. Collection development staff should be the first line of defense, ascertaining before accepting the gift whether the material will actually enhance the collection, turning away that which is unneeded. Even though decisions on acceptance of gifts and interactions with donors are typically not the duty of the acquisitions staff, often the resulting processing burdens are, and too seldom are staff provisions made to deal with these tasks. If acquisitions staff are drawn into dealing with donors, they should be aware of the legal requirements for documentation that must be met if the donor wishes to claim a tax deduction on the gift [104].

With their clientele's understandable emphasis on up-to-date information, health sciences libraries may find the most common gifts especially exasperating—those emanating from the retiring staff physician or faculty member, or family survivors cleaning out long-occupied offices. Except for items that might be added as institutional or local history material, or journal issues needed to fill in gaps, the outdated monographs and duplicate journals common in such collections will seldom be deemed useful. All medical libraries face a similar problem and avail themselves of several options of disposing of the excess material [105]. Book sales, a give-away table, or the dumpster are among the disposal options, which are discussed fully in later chapters.

Acquisition By Exchange

Exchanges, in which one institution's or one country's publications are exchanged for another's, are usually not a major component of acquisitions in health sciences libraries. However, libraries may find it advantageous to exchange, for political or other reasons, reports, newsletters, house organs, or current acquisitions lists with libraries of similar size or related by some other affinity. To enter into a specific exchange is usually a collection development decision, but acquisitions staff may be asked to formalize the arrangements, monitor the exchange, and conduct the correspondence after the initial agreement.

Acquisition By License

Electronic formats are frequently acquired through licensing rather than outright purchase. Acquisition through licensing is fundamentally different from acquisition by purchase, in that the library does not receive unrestricted ownership of the material; it only assumes the right to use the material or information for a specific period of time under specified conditions. From a library's operational point of view, licensing agreements tend to be more restrictive and protective of the publisher or producer than is the copyright law [106].

One special acquisitions task is to obtain a copy of the licensing agreement, make certain that it is brought to the attention of those who can decide if the library is willing and legally able to abide by the agreement's rules, and then follow that agreement. Often this means that as updates of the product are received, the outdated version must be returned to the producer or destroyed. Also acquisitions staff should be trained not to unpack materials received on license until the authorized person has reviewed and approved the license, because some software producers construe the opening of the diskette package as agreement to the license. This area of acquisitions by license is one that is expected to expand rapidly in the next few years, especially as libraries install local area networks allowing users online access from multiple locations [107].

Receiving, Paying for, and Routing Materials

Acquisitions staff need to document receipt of all materials for later reference. The receiving process includes both matching the item-in-hand with the existing record, to assure that what was ordered or expected has indeed been provided, and updating the order record to show date of receipt and other information. Of course, when no order record exists because material has been obtained through an approval or blanket order plan, or was received as a gift or exchange, creating the order record becomes the first part of the receiving process.

In the dynamic world of serials check-in, surprises and exceptions are expected. Journals cease and are born, titles change and merge. The acquisitions staff are expected to catch these changes and bring them to the attention of the appropriate person, be that the head of the unit or a serials cataloger. The staff members who receive and pay for serials should also be alert for excessive or unexpected price increases, and should report such to the personnel empowered to make collection development decisions.

Reviewing invoices, approving them for payment, and debiting the appropriate funds require thorough training, close attention to detail, a generous measure of good sense, and close supervision. The quality of the integrated library system's accounting module can make life easier or harder for the acquisitions staff, as can the link between the library and the institutional accounting system. But in any case, only meticulous attention to well-designed procedures can make invoice paying proceed efficiently and accurately.

Materials going through acquisitions processing have different priorities and different destinations. Once serials are checked in they need to be routed to particular reading areas, individuals, or departments. Some titles may demand rush handling; the *New England Journal of Medicine* and *JAMA* should be available to readers as quickly as possible after their stories have hit the nightly news. Books are normally sent to cataloging, but may need to be rush handled or tagged for a special final location; CD-ROMs may need to be directed to the systems staff for processing and loading. Mishaps and mistakes in these mundane routing tasks cause perhaps the most frequent and serious complaints brought against the acquisitions staff, because they are immediately visible and disruptive to good public service.

Claiming

Not all ordered materials arrive as expected. Especially serials, where one title may generate twelve or twenty-four deliveries a year, are prone to unpredictable lapses. As a result, one of the most important and time-consuming acquisitions challenges is to track overdue orders and claim items that are not delivered within a reasonable time span.

Computer library systems have made this task easier and more automatic—or should have; the quality of an automated technical processing program will be judged in large part by the abilities of its claiming module. For example, a claim flag or notice should be produced for books that have not been received after an interval which can be set by the library, and which might differ for domestic and overseas orders. For serials, the system should be able to identify skipped issues and produce an automatic claim; and, even more desirable, the system should be able to detect overdue issues, based on the title's publication frequency.

Tracking Expenditures and Fund Balances

The actual issuance of payment for materials received may or may not be carried out within the library. But the steps leading up to authorizing payment, including allocating charges to the appropriate fund and being able to account for expenditures from all funds, are among the most exacting acquisitions tasks. Libraries differ as to whether monies for materials are kept in one fund or are divided among separate funds according to various schemes, such as by publication format, disciplines to be served, or by the person(s) assigned responsibility to spend the monies. Special gifts or endowment monies are usually kept separate from institutional funds.

Staff need to understand clearly what funds are to be used for what materials; they should be meticulous in debiting the correct fund; and, through the automated system or by printed records, they should, when required, be able to produce annual lists for donors or trustees of what was bought on special funds. Librarians unfamiliar with standard accounting practices should refer to a basic treatment of the subject [108]. The sophistication of the automated accounting module will dictate the actual procedures for tracking expenditures, checking and releasing invoices, and authorizing payment. Accounting reports, such as monthly ledgers, in print or online, need to be checked. Were charges appropriate? Are outstanding encumbrances reasonable? Were the correct funds used? Do library records agree with those in the central accounting department? Are various fund balances sufficient to last through the year? If expenditures and budgeted allocations start to diverge, it is an acquisitions responsibility to alert appropriate staff.

The greatest demand for timely and accurate tracking of expenditures occurs near the end of the institution's fiscal year cycle, especially if, as is usually the case, all funds must be expended by a certain date or be lost. Unfortunately staffing levels are almost never expandable to meet such peak load demands [109]. Close cooperation between collection development and acquisitions operations can even out the flow of orders throughout the year and prevent the need for year-end panic buying. However, only the best of fund accounting systems can ease the unavoidable pressure of releasing within a short time as many invoices as possible, and providing up-to-date fund information. A loss of funds can be prevented by understanding those institutional policies governing year-end funds, such as what happens to encumbered funds and uncommitted balances.

Other Acquisitions Functions

Withdrawals

Although the decision about what to withdraw is properly a collection development decision, the attendant processing tasks are frequently handled by acquisitions personnel. For serials, holdings records must be adjusted, and all types of material normally require a "withdrawn" marking before they are removed from the library. Guilt, fear of public opinion, and possible legal issues can arise from discarding library materials; it happens very rarely, but acquisitions as well as collection development librarians may become embroiled in questions of appropriate disposition of institutional property [110].

Replacements

In the health sciences library, the replacement of lost or damaged monographs may not be a busy operation, since currency of materials is so important. Book and media selectors generally favor the purchase of an additional new work over the replacement of one that is more than two or three years old. Most of the direct replacements are for lost or stolen texts of recent vintage and thus do not pose an acquisitions challenge, but there may be an occasional out-of-print classic that stretches the acquisitions librarian's knowledge of the reprint and second-hand trade.

In contrast, replacing serial issues to ensure unbroken runs of important titles may be a major operation in a large library. This activity demands dealing with a variety of sources, from dealers to reprint houses to exchanges. The acquisitions librarian must be aware of possible sources and should do a cost-benefit analysis to evaluate them. An evaluation should consider factors such as staff time necessary to use each source and usual speed of service, in addition to the actual price charged for each issue.

Replacement of print materials by microforms is an often-used alternative. In addition, availability of the material in CD-ROM or even full-text online form must be considered more and more frequently. The acceptability of such media in place of print depends heavily upon the amount and type of illustrations in the original and the quality of the available reproduction equipment. There should be clear library policies as to what replacement medium will be acceptable for each category of titles.

Binding and Preservation

Knowing when a serials volume is ready for binding, what issues it should contain, and what supplements should accompany it, are challenging bindery preparation functions which require close coordination with other serial control procedures. Picking up the correct issues from current shelves; putting them in order and checking for completeness; designating the desired cover material and the appropriate text to be stamped on the spine; and updating internal processing records are some of the major tasks of the bindery function. When the bindery preparation unit is administratively separate from serials acquisitions, close cooperation and effective communication between them are essential.

Binding and rebinding are preservation means of choice for current serials, paperback books, and damaged hardcover volumes. Acquisitions staff are also involved in preservation when the means of preservation is replacement of the item, whether in the same or alternative format. In such cases sources of availability for the title must be sought and, when found, the functions of ordering and payment carried out. The ALA *Acquisition Guidelines* series includes a guide to preservation in acquisitions processing [111].

Document Delivery and Interlibrary Borrowing

It seems strange to speak of interlibrary borrowing and document delivery in a chapter on acquisitions. Yet these activities are more frequently being spoken of as a logical extension of traditional acquisitions procedures, since they are both involved with ordering, receiving, and paying for information materials for library users [112-115]. In this view, it does not really matter whether the needed materials are procured by buying the title, by borrowing it, or by obtaining in reproduction just the small part the user needs. Because these activities are still more frequently discussed than actually performed under the rubric of "acquisitions," their treatment will be deferred until the final section of this chapter.

Statistical Reports

Since acquisitions activities are so highly process oriented, there are many items and records and processes to count. Such statistics are important both to provide a picture of the library's collection and to quantify the work output of the department. Number of orders placed; number of volumes and titles received by purchase or gift or exchange; number of serial issues checked in; new, ceased, cancelled and withdrawn serial titles in the system — these are examples of what the acquisitions staff, or the automated system, may be required to count. The more management and workflow numbers can be derived from the computer system, the better. But in either case—for manual or automated statistics—the same questions must be asked: Are the data necessary? Why is it desirable to know the data? Are only similar things counted under each category? Is what is being counted clearly defined?

Acquisitions Automation

Automation of three areas of the acquisitions process has had a profound impact on the internal organization of acquisitions and on its connections inside and outside the institution. These areas are the creation and updating of the bibliographic record, the creation and updating of the financial record, and data transmission and exchange pertaining to both of these. Reorganization and realignment of these functions frequently occurs as a concomitant to the automation of processing tasks, or of change from one automated system to another. Even though thoughtful authors point out that automation should be no more than a handmaiden, in reality, automation drives organization.

The bibliographic record connects the various divisions of a library and its users. As long as information about selection, ordering, and cataloging of materials was kept in discrete paper files, territoriality and separation between the departments controlling each of those files arose naturally. As soon as the files disappeared and a single machine-readable record took their place—a record equally accessible to all personnel and users—cooperation between staffs necessarily ensued [116].

All technical services staff now have an equal stake in producing a complete, accurate record that will not cause unwanted duplication, that will state unambiguously which items have been ordered and received, and that will stand as a reliable base on which to add further information. Public services and users benefit from this combined effort, with an unobstructed view of what is on the shelf, what is on order, and what is waiting in the back room.

The importance of appropriate fiscal control and accurate financial accounting has been previously discussed. The capabilities of the automated library system determine most directly how efficiently and correctly these tasks will be accomplished. A good book fund accounting system will provide built-in verifications and safeguards to prevent many errors. By not wasting the considerable time needed to hunt down and correct totals that do not balance and invoices that have not been paid, such an automated accounting system saves staff time and improves relations with suppliers.

Electronic data transfer in place of rekeying has the greatest potential for cutting error rates and increasing both speed and efficiency in technical processing. Within the institution, links for automatic data transfer between library and accounting office are desirable [117]. External connections to national bibliographic utilities and vendor systems (and an interface to map and translate data formats between computers) can be used to download bibliographic information and send orders, claims, and payments with a minimum investment of human effort [118].

In a world of networks, gateways, and the virtual library, the environment for acquisitions tasks is changing forever [119]. Even as many libraries are finally achieving their automation goal of a fully integrated library system, technological innovations may once again tip the balance in favor of a modular approach, accommodating closer links with external vendor systems [120]. It is obvious that acquisitions librarians must learn all they can about telecommunications and networking, and they must become actively involved in network planning for their institutions.

Finally, something should be said about the cost of automating acquisitions tasks. Contrary to the early dreams of vast personnel savings stemming from automation, experience has led to a different awareness. "Innovation and technology improve the cost/efficiency ratio by raising the efficiency not by lowering the cost" [121]. During the years of initial implementation of an integrated automated library system, costs may, in fact, go up [122]. The increased productivity and opportunity for staff reduction that automation brings to acquisition functions has often been offset by the costs of maintaining the automated system—without even considering its initial capital cost. To the equation, however, must be added the intangible yet real benefit that more service and information is being provided users than was ever possible in preautomation days.

Acquisitions Personnel

One of the few "professional" positions in a library for which no standard of education is widely agreed upon is that of head of the acquisitions section. All concur that reference librarians should hold an MLS degree (or equivalent), although it is acceptable to use paraprofessionals for some public desk duties; and cataloging is universally divided into original cataloging, certainly done by professionals, and copy cataloging, acceptably performed by paraprofessionals. But must a professional librarian head the acquisitions operation, or can other training and background substitute for the library degree?

Those aspects of acquisitions that point to a need for library school training are the ones concerned with the bibliographic record and with establishing the unique identity of a published item. The acquisitions head guides staff in searching bibliographic databases to identify and verify information perhaps sketchily supplied by other staff or users. The same person provides the training that allows downloading from a national utility of the one best record, and knows what nuances of the MARC record must be present to satisfy catalogers.

But these bibliographic skills are only part of the strengths needed for running a successful acquisitions program. Other professional elements concern planning and managing operations in harmony with broader library goals, and the ability to adapt to changes in the information environment. Can these skills be learned only in library school or will other schooling, experience, and on-the-job training suffice? Where does one best learn about accounting practices and budget forecasting, how does one become familiar with publishing practices and purchasing rules, or gain knowledge about computer programs and telecommunications? The answers to these questions remain unresolved.

There is a realistic concern about job satisfaction for a professionally trained head of the acquisitions operation. A common solution is to split assignments for the librarian between collection development or cataloging, and acquisitions. Other libraries head their acquisitions departments with a senior-grade nonlibrarian, experienced enough to manage the administrative and business aspects of the job and already familiar with the bibliographic aspects through training and experience. Both these models have been used in health sciences libraries. The nonlibrarian head may report to the head of collection development or cataloging, or may function as an independent department head. The issue of whether acumen in the business or the bibliographic aspects of the job should determine choice of a department head is complicated by the fact that few library schools teach a course in acquisitions, and most acquisitions librarians state that their learning was done on the job [123-126]. Those librarians who have found their way to acquisitions work agreed on what they wish they had been taught in library school:

- A fundamental understanding of the economics of publishing, including pricing policies and marketing techniques.

- Instruction in the business practices of publishing and serials and book vending.

- Accounting techniques.

- Purchasing ethics.

- Skills in evaluating various methods of material procurement.

- Administrative techniques.

- Personnel management.

The library assistants or, in the small library, the librarian, who will be processing acquired materials need basic clerical skills, skill in quality control and data verification, computer literacy, and some accounting skills. Such training is usually provided on the job, one-on-one; large university library systems, however, may hold occasional basic training classes for new assistants in all library branches.

In an academic setting it may be efficient to use college students for some acquisitions tasks—for example, those which need little training, such as opening mail, date stamping serials issues, and security treating materials. Alternatively, tasks which need high concentration and are best done for only an hour or two at a time, such as serials check-in, can be assigned to students. Students can also provide the muscle power which is often needed for receiving books and moving gifts. Since the student option is not available in all library settings, there may be a desire to substitute volunteers for students. A great divergence of opinion exists as to the use of volunteer labor in libraries [127-128]. In the acquisitions setting it is important to remember that whatever the classification of the persons performing acquisitions tasks, they must be well trained and motivated. Because of the detail-specific nature of acquisitions work, except for the most simple and intermittent tasks, occasional volunteers are not a useful solution.

The Present and the Future of Acquisitions

How to Stay Alive in the Present

Libraries of all sizes are affected by the same realities: shrinking budgets, rising costs, expanding information sources and, for health sciences libraries, a radically changing health care environment [129-131]. The hospital library is under especially strong pressure to prove its effectiveness and efficiency [132-134].

Under such strained circumstances it behooves libraries to conduct their acquisitions operations in the most cost-effective manner possible. Issues of cost control in acquisitions management have been well documented in the literature [135-136]. Optimum use of automation, and cutting unnecessary operations to lower personnel costs, are obvious internal measures to pursue. The acquisitions librarian can take steps to ensure that vendor charges are competitive by seeking alternative vendor proposals on a regular basis. Simplifying an approval plan profile by eliminating minor exceptions may garner a higher discount rate. Shifting subscriptions to provide a better mix of domestic and foreign journals to be supplied by one serials vendor may result in a lower service fee percentage. Frank discussion with book and serials vendors and an understanding of their business can bring about savings in these business interactions.

The acquisitions librarian is powerless to influence the high price of health sciences publications, but even in this area cost-saving measures are possible, such as taking advantage of prepublication promotions and obtaining early-payment discounts from subscription vendors. The problem with these approaches is that they may go against rules set by purchasing departments, which dictate that goods must be paid for and delivered in the same fiscal year. Sometimes logical persuasion will demonstrate the potential savings to accounting personnel and will allow contravention of such general policies.

It seems regrettable but true that "...acquisitions librarians cannot assume that their professional colleagues in the library possess even the most rudimentary understanding and appreciation for acquisitions work" [137]. To thrive, acquisitions librarians need to educate their colleagues; they need to convince them of their worth by contributing to the mission and goals of the library; they need to further their professional standing by conducting research into publishing, the book trade, and enhanced performance in their own areas of expertise; and they need to publish their ideas on how better to address the library's new missions.

How to Thrive in the Future

The changing role of the library and the librarian has been a recurring theme at library meetings for years, including those of the Medical Library Association and its regional chapters. The reasons these roles are changing are, first, that publishing is changing—the production and distribution of information are following new patterns—and second, technology, in terms of computing power, electronic storage, and telecommunications is improving at increasing rates. In other words, technology has affected both the format and the dissemination of information [138-139].

Up to now librarians have seen their job as managing the containers of information; now librarians must move toward dealing with the content of the containers, the information itself. Knowledge bases, expert systems, and interactive simulations are examples of new forms of information being sought out with increasing frequency [140]. The acquisitions operation, charged with obtaining the information the library and its users need, will be strongly affected by these developments. To respond effectively, careful consideration must be given to emerging trends—trends in how information will be disseminated, how and what will be acquired, and how the new technologies can help.

Access and Ownership

Acquisitions, as defined at the beginning of this chapter, includes the acquiring of packets of information, whether by purchase, gift, exchange, or by license. The visionaries of the library profession agree that a variety of converging trends are leading libraries away from outright purchase of all needed materials towards renting, leasing, or contracting for access to some of them. Acquisitions staff are already beginning to deal with these changes, as they sign licensing agreements for CD-ROM titles and monitor access charges for commercial electronic journals. They must prepare for an increasingly broad spectrum of acquisition strategies, including licensing, borrowing, and article-level acquisition.

Ross Atkinson has described a new role for the acquisitions librarian as change agent. He sees all information services divided into delivery and mediation, delivery being the shifting of physical information packets amongst locations, and mediation being the provision of assistance in the use of that information. Acquisitions, circulation, and interlibrary loan departments have the primary responsibilities for delivery, and must plan for the new requirements of a networked environment. In the setting of new publication methods and transfers, a key role can be played by the staff with the most understanding of the processes and economics of publication

— that is, the acquisitions staff—if it can undergo the necessary transformation [141].

New terms for acquisitions budgets emerged in the literature in the last two decades. From "book budget" the term changed to "materials budget" when microforms and audiovisuals became a library presence. Now there is a change again, to "information resources budget" [142], as libraries consolidate budgets for all forms of information delivery. New pricing formulas for information products are also emerging. The trend is clearly toward usage-based pricing, with licensing agreements for access to digitized information taking the place of subscriptions to successive printed information [143].

Negotiation of licenses can become complex when questions of local area networks, simultaneous users, or simultaneous workstations must be clarified. Because they are partly technology-dependent, such negotiations need to include systems staff; and because the convenience of users must be balanced against the cost of various modes of delivery, the public services head or even director of the library will need to be involved in licensing decisions. But without question, the acquisitions department is the logical center of the negotiations and the group that will finalize the agreement, document it on the appropriate computer record, and arrange for payment [144].

Organizational Realignments

At a 1992 ALA midwinter ALCTS meeting, these definitions for expanded acquisitions functions were quoted:

> Buying would include all purchases of information, whether it is in a traditional format or takes the form of an access service....It would also include the bibliographic verification for all materials...[it] would also include borrowing, which means this unit would acquire both permanent and temporary acquisitions. Borrowing would include what is currently the interlibrary-loan activity in most libraries. The third method of acquisitions is leasing of information. Most acquisition units now handle leasing of books, but few handle the leasing of electronic files, which would be the majority of this activity. Another part of this activity will be the handling of licensing agreements, which are becoming a more significant factor, particularly in many nonprint formats [145].

This ALA group, just as Atkinson proposed, charges acquisitions personnel with providing users with access to all information; that includes the "just-in-time" access furnished by interlibrary loan or document delivery as well as the more traditional "just-in-case" purchases. There is consensus at least among science librarians, who have experienced the worst of journal price increases, that libraries' rate of acquisitions for the general collection will decrease and the rate of information obtained for specific end users, either via the library or bypassing it completely, will increase [146]. Academic health sciences libraries are discussing internal organizational changes that would help to put more emphasis and focus on the user [147]; allying acquisitions functions with document delivery thus begins to make real operational sense [148].

Some jarring adjustments may be necessary during the transition period when the overwhelming majority of acquisitions efforts still deal with traditional print purchases, but the shift to new areas is being made. Organizational realignments within the library may temporarily imperil the efficiency of the workflow, but technical services departments must make sure to maintain their present collective strength as they align with new partners for the future.

Connectivity

The connectivity that ties a single workstation to a worldwide network of institutions and individuals is already an established reality to an amazing degree [149]. Acquisitions staff can interact with a complete range of databases beyond their own institution. They can check in journals on a remote database, see what dealers have in stock, and order books online. Information between selectors and those who order flows back and forth via e-mail or within the library's integrated online system [150]. By 2001, acquisitions and collection development departments should be linked by computer to all appropriate library and commercial sources [151]. Libraries may be able to realize a savings in telecommunication costs by allowing vendors to dial in to the library's computer for uploading and downloading of order data [152]. The increasing availability of vendor computers on the Internet should also bring down costs and facilitate library-vendor connectivity.

Most exciting for acquisitions personnel and potentially most useful is electronic data interchange (EDI) between publishers, vendors and libraries. "EDI…is the last significant area in which technical services librarians can expect to achieve significant economies. The major wins from automation in cataloging and acquisitions/serials control have been made, save what EDI can do" [153]. EDI is not like sending e-mail messages or files, which must be received, translated, and then fed into the local system. Nor is it like loading data from tape. EDI is "the exchange of unambiguous information in highly structured standard electronic formats suitable for satisfying business needs of trading partners, across industries, and without human interpretation" [154]. Thus the data elements of an invoice, an order, or a claim—which now must be keyed and rekeyed, potentially introducing errors and delays—could be transmitted from computer to computer according to strict standards. When EDI is fully implemented by libaries and vendors, orders, invoices, dispatch date, claims, and claims responses will shuttle seemlessly and transparently between vendors and purchasers.

Emerging Standards

Widely agreed upon standards of organizing information have long been a success story of librarianship and a source of strength and unity for the profession. Few coding schemes, for example, have proved as flexible and universal as the MARC format. For the new methods of packaging and distributing information, new standards are in the process of emerging, although the birth process is incomplete [155-156]. "NISO + BISAC + SISAC + Z39 + X12 = CHAOS" was the title of an ALA preconference on standards for the acquisition of library materials, and a warning of what acquisitions librarians will have to forge, assimilate, and build upon in the next few years [157].

Standards are obviously necessary to code data beyond the bibliographic record, so that it may be stored, enhanced, and transmitted from computer to computer, from vendor to library to national network. A recent list of the kinds of standards needed to develop scholarly communication tools and networks is illuminating for its breadth:

- Data creation—content.
- Data structure—storage—handling.
- Data identification—representation—display.
- Data transfer—distribution—production.
- Data integrity.
- Operating systems.
- Access systems—user interface.
- Communication system—protocols.
- Connectivity.
- Navigation (and directory services).

- Tracking.

- Archiving—preservation [158].

The present and future array of acquisitions functions will need to use all these standards, so that receipt of serial issues can be acknowledged, missing issues claimed, payment transmitted, orders specified, and messages forwarded to the right person, electronically and with minimal human intervention. However, much development and testing remains to be carried out before today's communication formats and data interchange standards are ready for the electronic acquisition age.

Sorting Out the Soup

Acquisitions departments will survive if they will perform their present tasks better by exploiting the potentials of new technologies. They will thrive if they can become part of the information delivery systems that will support scholarly communication as it evolves. As such, they can continue to fulfill their basic role, providing access to information, however that information is produced, packaged, or disseminated.

This same thought was more poetically and forcefully expressed thus:

> Let us start outside the library, in the world of publishing and information distribution, knowledge and opinion brokers, and of information consumers. It is a world we can see as "Information Soup" on the one hand. And on the other, it is a world of the "Information Soup-Hungry."...
>
> Libraries' first dimension is the interpretation of Information Soup for indentification/selection/contracting-to-get. It includes direct contact with the unadorned reality of Information Soup to determine what's out there (identification) and whether (selection) and how (contracting) to get it into the library. This is "acquisitions" in the most inclusive sense of the word....
>
> [In the] electronic age, the future of acquisitions, defined in the broad, first-dimension sense, seems to me to be guaranteed for as long as libraries exist. The First Dimension is vital to making the Information Soup unchaotic enough that it can be selected, labeled, and served;...But we...will often be utterly transparent to the Soup-Hungry and to those working in the third dimension [i.e., public services]....Modern acquisitions people I see as having the task of legitimizing, codifying, authorizing, and enabling (through

payments, behind-the-scenes money management, and contract and license controls) those other dimensions [159].

Finally, a sanity-preserving motto for acquisitions staff during the changes of the near future, something another library luminary quoted from Samuel Beckett: "Ever tried. Ever failed. Never mind. Try again. Fail better" [160].

References

1. Atkinson R. The acquisitions librarian as change agent in the transition to the electronic library. Libr Res Tech Serv 1992 Jan;36(1):7-20.

2. Ogburn JL. The value of acquisitions in the library of the future. Libr Acquis Pract Theory 1991 Fall;15(3):355-8.

3. Kronick DA, Bowden VM. Health science library materials: acquisitions. In: Darling L, Bishop D, Colaianni LA, eds. Handbook of medical library practice. 4th ed. v.2. Technical services in health science libraries. Chicago: Medical Library Association, 1983:93-138.

4. Hewitt JA. On the nature of acquisitions. Libr Res Tech Serv 1989 Apr;33(2):105-22.

5. Schmidt KA. Please, Sir, I want some more: a review of the literature of acquisitions, 1990. Libr Res Tech Serv 1991 Jul; 35(3):245-54.

6. Boissonnas C. Desperately seeking status: acquisition librarians in academic libraries. Libr Acquis Pract Theory 1991 Fall;15(3):349-354.

7. Hewitt, op. cit., 105.

8. O'Neill AL. Evaluating the success of acquisitions departments: a literature review. Libr Acquis Pract Theory 1992 Fall;16(3):206-16.

9. Maxwell J. Whether it is better to be loved or feared: acquisition librarianship as Machiavelli might have described it. Libr Acquis Pract Theory 1992 Summer;16(2):113-7.

10. American Library Association. Bookdealer-Library Relations Committee. Guidelines for handling library orders for in-print monographic publications. Chicago: American Library Association, 1973. (Acquisition guidelines no. 1).

11. Bosch S. Guide to selecting and acquiring CD-ROMs, software and other electronic publications. Chicago: American Library Association, 1994. (Acquisition guidelines no. 9).

12. Miller HS. Managing acquisitions and vendor relations: a how-to-do-it manual. New York: Neal-Schuman, 1992.

13. Magrill RM, Corbin J. Acquisitions management and collection development in libraries. 2d ed. Chicago: American Library Association, 1989.

14. Cenzer PS, Gozzi CI, eds. Evaluating acquisitions and collection management. New York: Haworth Press, 1991.

15. Lee SH, ed. Issues in acquisitions: programs and evaluation. Ann Arbor, MI: Pierian Press, 1984.

16. Coffey JR, ed. Operational costs in acquisitions. New York: Haworth Press, 1990.

17. Pitkin GM, ed. Cost-effective technical services: how to track, manage, and justify internal operations. New York: Neal-Schuman, 1989.

18. Schmidt KA, ed. Understanding the business of library acquisitions. Chicago: American Library Association, 1990.

19. Katz B, ed. Vendors and library acquisitions. New York: Haworth Press, 1991.

20. Genaway DC, ed. Acquisitions '90: Conference on Acquisitions, Budgets, and Collections. Canfield, OH: Genaway, 1990.

21. Godden IP, ed. Library technical services: operations and management. 2d ed. San Diego: Academic Press, 1991.

22. Gorman M, ed. Technical services today and tomorrow. Englewood, CO: Libraries Unlimited, 1990.

23. Leonhardt TW, ed. Technical services in libraries: systems and applications. Greenwich, CT: JAI Press, 1992. (Foundations in library and information science, vol. 25).

24. Racine D, ed. Managing technical services in the 1990's. New York: Haworth Press, 1991.

25. Basch NB, McQueen J. Buying serials: a how-to-do-it manual for librarians. New York: Neal-Schuman, 1990.

26. Tuttle M, Cook JG, eds. Advances in serials management. Greenwich, CT: JAI Press, 1988.

27. Morse D, ed. Biomedical library acquisitions bulletin (BLAB). dmorse@hsc.usc.edu.

28. Cook E, ed. ACQNET. acqnet-1@listserv.appstate.edu

29. ALCTS network news (AN2). listserv@uicvm.cc.uic.edu:subscribe ALCTS.

30. Tuttle M, ed. Newsletter on serials pricing issues. listserv@unc.edu: subscribe prices [name].

31. Brandon AN, Hill DR. Selected list of books and journals for the small medical library. Bull Med Libr Assoc, 1995 Apr;83(2):151-75.

32. Hafner AW, Filipowicz AB, Whitely WP. Computers in medicine: liability issues for physicians. Int J Clin Monit Comput 1989 Jul;6(3):185-94.

33. Tomaiuolo NG. Does malpractice make MEDLINE mandatory? MD Comput 1992 Nov-Dec;9(6):346-7.

34. Dorsch JL, Frasca MA, Wilson ML, Tomsic ML. A multidisciplinary approach to information and critical appraisal instruction. Bull Med Libr Assoc 1990 Jan;78(1):38-44.

35. Advisory Panel for Scientific Publications. The cost-effectiveness of scientific publications. Pub Res Q 1992 Fall;8(3):72-91.

36. Cummings AM, et al. University libraries and scholarly communication; a study prepared for The Andrew W. Mellon Foundation. Washington, DC: The Association of Research Libraries, 1992.

37. Brown GJ. The business of scholarly journal publishing. In: Schmidt KA. Understanding the business of library acquisitions. Chicago: American Library Association, 1990:33-48.

38. Perrault AH. The shrinking national collection: a study of the effects of the diversion of funds from monographs to serials on the monograph collections of research libraries. Libr Acquis Pract Theory 1994 Spring;18(1):3-22.

39. Okerson A. Of making many books there is no end. In: Report of the ARL Serials Project. Washington, DC: The Association of Research Libraries, 1989:2-10.

40. Byrd GD. An economic 'commons' tragedy for research libraries: scholarly journal publishing and pricing trends. Coll Res Libr 1990 May;51(3):184-95.

41. Hamaker C. Library serials budgets: publishers and the twenty percent effect. Libr Acquis Pract Theory 1988 Summer;12(2):211-9.

42. Fleishauer C, McSweeney MG. Acquisition's role of facilitator between the demand of various library units, also to balance needs of vendor, publisher, library. In: Cenzer PS, Gozzi CI, eds. Evaluating acquisitions and collection management. New York: Haworth Press, 1991.

43. Melkin A. Publishers, vendors, libraries: troublesome issues in the triangle. In: Schmidt KA. Understanding the business of library acquisitions. Chicago: American Library Association, 1990:21-32.

44. Alessi D. Up the elevator: an examination of approval plan inflation and its impact on libraries. In: Lee SH, ed. Acquisitions, budgets and material costs: issues and approaches. New York: Haworth Press, 1988:49-52.

45. Leonhardt TW. The importance of approval plans when budgets are lean. In: Lee SH, ed. Acquisitions, budgets and material costs: issues and approaches. New York: Haworth Press, 1988:1-13.

46. Coffey JR. Contracts and ethics in library acquisitions: the expressed and the implied. In: Strauch K, Strauch B, eds. Legal and ethical issues in acquisitions. New York: Haworth Press, 1990:95-110.

47. Marsh C. Payment ethics: librarians as consumers. In: Schmidt KA. Understanding the business of library acquisitions. Chicago: American Library Association, 1990:299-312.

48. Lynden FC. Prices and discounts. Libr Acquis Pract Theory 1988 Summer;12(2):255-8.

49. Mosher PH. Waiting for Godot: rating approval service vendors. In: Spyers-Duran P, Mann T, Jr., eds. Shaping library collections for the 1980s. Phoenix, AZ: Oryx Press, 1980:159-66.

50. Presley RL. Firing an old friend, painful decisions: the ethics between librarians and vendors. Libr Acquis Pract Theory 1993 Spring;17(1):53-9.

51. Barker JW. Random vendor assignment in vendor performance evaluation. Libr Acquis Pract Theory 1986 Summer;10(2):265-80.

52. Dannelly GN. The "E's" of vendor selection: an archetype for selection, evaluation, and sustenance. In: Schmidt KA. Understanding the business of library acquisitions. Chicago: American Library Association, 1990:109.

53. Ivins O. The development of criteria and methodologies for evaluation of the performance of monographic and serials vendors. Adv Ser Manage 1988;2:185-212.

54. Katz, op. cit.

55. Miller, op. cit.

56. Schmidt KA. Understanding the business of library acquisitions, op. cit., 1990:95-164.

57. Fisher W. A brief history of library-vendor relations since 1950. Libr Acquis Pract Theory 1993 Spring;17(1):61-9.

58. Shirk GM. Contract acquisitions: change, technology, and the new library/vendor partnership. Libr Acquis Pract Theory 1993 Summer;17(2):145-53.

59. Gorman M. Ethics in acquisitions. Reported in the ALCTS Acquisitions Administrators discussion group. Libr Acquis Pract Theory 1992 Winter;16(4):417-29.

60. Bushing MC. Acquisitions ethics: the evolution of models for hard times. Libr Acquis Pract Theory 1993 Spring;17(1):47-52.

61. Lindsey JA. Appreciation and/or motivation — ethics and the library/vendor relationship. Technicalities 1984 May;4(5):12.

62. Goehner D. Vendor-library relations: the ethics of working with vendors. In: Schmidt KA. Understanding the business of library acquisitions. Chicago: American Library Association, 1990:137-51.

63. Pisciotta RA, ed. Librarian/vendor relations: a symposium. Special suppl. to Tech Trends (Technical Services Section) and Developments (Collection Development Section of the Medical Library Association) 1990:1-10.

64. Bazirjian R. The ethics of library discard practices. In: Strauch K., Strauch B, eds. Legal and ethical issues in acquisitions. New York: Haworth Press, 1990:135-146.

65. Carlson BA. Claiming periodicals: the "trembling balance" in the "feud of want and have". In: Strauch K. Legal and ethical issues in acquisitions. New York: Haworth Press, 1990:119-127.

66. Winters B. ALCTS Acquisition Section's membership meeting. ALCTS Network News 1993 Mar 26;5(18):1-2.

67. Barker JW. Integrating acquisitions: reorganization at the University of California, Berkeley. Libr Acquis Pract Theory 1992 Winter;16(4):355-60.

68. Bennett LL. Authority control at the order process: what do catalogers want, and do we care; the NOTIS environment—Loyola perspective. Libr Acquis Pract Theory 1992 Spring;16(1):71-4.

69. Davis TL. Blurring the lines in technical services. Libr Acquis Pract Theory 1993 Spring;17(1):85-7.

70. Dewey GL. Technical services reorganization at the University of Wisconsin-Madison: a subject-oriented approach. Libr Acquis Pract Theory 1992 Winter;16(4):373-7.

71. McCombs GM. Technical services in the 1990s: a process of convergent evolution. Libr Res Tech Serv 1992 Summer;36(2):135-48.

72. Niles J. Acquisitions and collection management reorganization: an exercise in crisis management. Libr Acquis Pract Theory 1992 Winter;16(4):379-82.

73. Ogburn JL. Organizing acquisitions: the Yale University experience. Libr Acquis Pract Theory 1992 Winter;16(4):367-72.

74. Wachel K, Shreeves E. An alliance between acquisitions and collection management. Libr Acquis Pract Theory 1992 Winter;16(4):383-9.

75. Corbin J. Technology and organizational change in libraries. Libr Acquis Pract Theory 1992 Winter;16(4):349-53.

76. McCombs, op. cit., 140.

77. Lowell GR, Sullivan M. Self-management in technical services: the Yale experience. Libr Adm Manage 1990 Jan;4(1):20-3.

78. Barker JW. Integrating acquisitions, op. cit., 356.

79. Corbin, op. cit., 351.

80. Trujillo TF. Acquisitions administration requirements: current and future. Presented at Acquisition Administrators' discussion group, June 25, 1990, as reported by JL Flowers. Libr Acquis Pract Theory 1991 Spring;15(1):131.

81. Trujillo TF. Perspectives on acquisitions librarianship: today and tomorrow. In: Leonhardt TW, ed. Technical services in libraries: systems and applications. Greenwich, CT: JAI Press, 1992: 197-205.

82. Wachel, op. cit., 384-7.

83. Jasper RP, Treadwell JB. Reorganizing collections and technical services: staffing is key. Libr Acquis Pract Theory 1992 Winter;16(4):361-6.

84. Wachel, op. cit., 388.

85. Dewey, op. cit., 376.

86. Hoadley IB, Corbin J. Up the beanstalk: an evolutionary organizational structure for libraries. Am Libr 1990 Jul-Aug;21(7):676-8.

87. Bazirjian R. Automation and technical services organization. Libr Acquis Pract Theory 1993 Spring;17(1):73-7.

88. Somers SW. Life in a gold fish bowl: or the changing nature of acquisitions work in an integrated online environment. In: Dykeman A, Katz B, eds. Automated acquisitions: issues for the present and future. New York: Haworth Press, 1989.

89. Heinz R, Ogburn J. Communicating voucher information to the accounting department from automated library systems. Against the Grain 1991 Jan;3(1):36-7.

90. Jarvis WE. Interactions between acquisition system expenditure reports and university financial services payment systems: WLN Acquis to WSU's PAPR. Libr Acquis Pract Theory 1992 Winter;16(4):405-10.

91. Barker JW. The University of California, Berkeley library: in search of the optimal link with campus accounting. Libr Acquis Pract Theory 1992 Winter;16(4):411-4.

92. Bazirjian R, Randall LE. The accounting office interface: Syracuse University. Libr Acquis Pract Theory 1992 Winter;16(4):393-403.

93. Hardy ED. Managing acquisitions finances. Libr Acquis Pract Theory 1992 Summer;16(2):183-4.

94. Hawks CP. Internal control, auditing, and the automated acquisitions system. J Acad Libr 1990 Nov;16(5):296-301.

95. Ibid., 298-9.

96. Magrill, op. cit., 117.

97. Magrill, op. cit., 213.

98. Schmidt KA. The business of acquisitions. In: Genaway, DC, ed. Acquisitions '90: Conference on Acquisitions, Budgets, and Collections. Canfield, OH: Genaway, 1990:35-8.

99. Grant J. Approval plans: the vendor as preselector. In: Schmidt KA. Understanding the business of library acquisitions. Chicago: American Library Association, 1990:153-64.

100. Kahin B. Information policy and the Internet: toward a public information infrastructure in the United States. Governm Publ Rev 1991 Sep/Oct;18(5):451-72.

101. Gersh D. Government electronic database proposed: Congressional legislation introduced to make government documents available to the public via computer. Editor Publisher 1992 Aug 1;125(31):10-11.

102. Ebersole JL. Competition, jobs, and information policy: the case for private-sector information services; U.S. patents. J Governm Inf 1994 Mar-Apr;21(2):83-104.

103. Plesser R. Competition and cost concerns: information as a commodity—fee vs. free; provider concerns. J Agric Food Inf 1994;2(1):35-6.

104. Clark M. Gifts and exchanges. In: Schmidt, KA. Understanding the business of library acquisitions. Chicago: American Library Association, 1990:167-85.

105. Cooper ER. Options for the disposal of unwanted donations. Bull Med Libr Assoc 1990 Oct;78(4):388-94.

106. Nissley M. CD-ROMs, licenses and librarians. In: Nissley M, Nelson NM, eds. CD-ROM licensing and copyright issues for libraries. Westport, CT: Meckler, 1990:1-17.

107. Davis TL. Acquisition of CD-ROM databases for local area networks. J Acad Libr 1993 May;19(2):68-71.

108. Kruger B. Basic acquisitions accounting. In: Schmidt KA. Understanding the business of library acquisitions. Chicago: American Library Association, 1990:261-85.

109. Hewitt, op. cit., 112.

110. Bazirjian R. The ethics of library discard practices. In: Strauch K, Strauch B, eds. Legal and ethical issues in acquisitions. New York: Haworth Press, 1990:135-46.

111. Hamilton MJ. Guide to preservation in acquisitions processing. Chicago: American Library Association, 1993. (Acquisition guidelines no. 8).

112. Gammon JA. Is there a future for acquisitions and document delivery: an introduction. Libr Acquis Pract Theory 1993 Fall;17(3):345-6.

113. Ray RL. A skeptics view of the future for combined acquisitions and document delivery. Libr Acquis Pract Theory 1993 Fall;17(3):347-51.

114. Branche Brown LC. Expert systems and document delivery in an automated acquisitions environment. Libr Acquis Pract Theory 1993 Fall;17(3):353-7.

115. Van Goethem J. Whether by byte or by tome, buying information is acquisitions. Libr Acquis Pract Theory 1993 Fall;17(3):359-62.

116. Jasper RP. Automating acquisitions and serials: synthesis from chaos. Libr Acquis Pract Theory 1993 Spring;17(1):79-84.

117. Van Goethem J. From the INNOPAC/UNIX to the IBM ES9000 mainframe via TCP/IP - the Duke University experience. Libr Acquis Pract Theory 1992 Winter;16(4):415-6.

118. Santosuosso J. Electronic data interchange (EDI) for libraries and publishers. Bull Amer Soc Inf Sci 1992 Oct-Nov;19(1):15-7.

119. Chamberlain CE. Technology for acquisitions and access: beyond the automated acquisitions system: introduction. Libr Acquis Pract Theory 1993 Summer;17(2):125.

120. Ray RL. The dis-integrating library system: effects of new technologies in acquisitions. Libr Acquis Pract Theory 1993 Summer;17(2):127-36.

121. Gorman M. The academic library in the year 2001: dream or nightmare or something in between? J Acad Libr 1991 Mar;17(1):4-9.

122. Phelps D. Cost impact on acquisitions in implementing an integrated online system. In: Coffey JR, ed. Operational costs in acquisitions. New York: Haworth Press, 1990:33-46.

123. Marcum DB. Acquisitions in the library school curriculum. Libr Acquis Pract Theory 1991 Winter;15(4):471-3.

124. Ogburn JL. Why we need acquisitions in the library science curriculum. Libr Acquis Pract Theory 1991 Winter;15(4):475-9.

125. Schmidt KA. Education for acquisitions: a history. Libr Res Tech Serv 1990 Apr;34(2):159-69.

126. Schmidt KA. The education of the acquisitions librarian: a survey of ARL acquisitions librarians. Libr Res Tech Serv 1991 Jan;35(1):7-22.

127. Chadbourne R. Volunteers in the library; both sides must give in order to get. Wilson Libr Bull 1993 Jun;67(10):26-7.

128. White HS. The double-edged sword of library volunteerism. Libr J 1993 Apr 15;118(7):66-7.

129. Messerle J. Health sciences libraries: strategies in an era of changing economics. Bull Med Libr Assoc 1987 Jan;75(1):27-33.

130. Glaser WA. The United States needs a health system like other countries. JAMA 1993 Aug 25;270(8):980-4.

131. Peterson MA. Political influence in the 1990s: from iron triangles to policy networks. J Health Polit Policy Law 1993 Summer;18(2):395-438.

132. American Hospital Association. Vision, values, viability: 1989/1990 environmental assessment. Chicago: American Hospital Association, 1989:60-1.

133. Stevens SR. Impact of changing health care economics on Michigan hospital libraries: report of a survey. Bull Med Libr Assoc 1990 Apr;78(2):140-5.

134. O'Donnell KP. The last word; no more "business as usual" for hospitals. Hosp Health Netw 1993 Jun 20;67(12):68.

135. Coffey, Operational costs, op. cit.

136. Boissonnas CM. Acquisitions cost study at Cornell University Library. In: Pitkin GM, ed. Cost-effective technical services: how to track, manage, and justify internal operations. New York: Neal-Schuman, 1989:69-78.

137. Hewitt, op. cit., 108.

138. Lucier RE. Toward a knowledge management environment: a strategic framework. Educom Rev 1992 Nov-Dec;27(6):24-31.

139. Lynch CA. The transformation of scholarly communication and the role of the library in the age of networked information. Serials Libr 1993;23(3/4):5-20.

140. Braude R. Impact of information technology on the role of health sciences librarians. Bull Med Libr Assoc 1993 Oct;81(4):408-13.

141. Atkinson, op. cit., 17.

142. Winters BA. Organizational models: introduction. Libr Acquis Pract Theory 1992 Winter;16(4):345-8.

143. Sabosik PE. Electronic subscriptions. Serials Libr 1991;19(3/4):59-70.

144. Nissley M. Rave new world: librarians and electronic acquisitions. Libr Acquis Pract Theory 1993 Summer;17(2):165-73.

145. Hoadley, op. cit., 677.

146. Goodran R. ALCTS ALMS Acquisitions Librarians/Vendors of Library Materials Discussion Group. Libr Acquis Pract Theory 1992 Winter;16(4):421.

147. Jacobson S. Reorganization: premises, processes, and pitfalls. Bull Med Libr Assoc 1994 Oct; 82(4):369-74.

148. Van Goethem, Whether by byte, op. cit., 361-2.

149. Wood MS, ed. CD-ROM implementation and networking in health sciences libraries. New York: Haworth Press, 1993.

150. Farkas DG, Su ST. Electronic order request submission at UF libraries: three pilot programs. Libr Acquis Pract Theory 1992 Fall;16(3):275-88.

151. Barker JW. Acquisitions and collection development: 2001. Libr Acquis Pract Theory 1988 Summer;12(2):243-8.

152. Kelly GJ. Exploring costs of electronically transmitting information between a library and a vendor. Inf Technol Libr 1990 Mar;9(1):53-65.

153. Barker J, quoted in Gammon JA. EDI and acquisitions: the future is now! An introduction. Libr Acquis Pract Theory 1994 Spring;18(1):113-4.

154. Schwartz FE. The EDI horizon: implementing an ANSI X12 pilot project at the Faxon Company. Serials Libr 1991; 19(3/4):39-57.

155. Blixrud JC. Webs that link libraries, librarians, and information: evolving technical standards for a networking age. Serials Libr 1993;23(3/4):43-59.

156. Landesman B. EDI standards for acquisitions: they're (just about) he-ere.... Libr Acquis Pract Theory 1994 Spring;18(1):119-21.

157. Winters BA. NISO + BISAC + SISAC + Z39 + X12 = CHAOS: an ALA preconference on standards for the acquisition of library materials. Libr Acquis Pract Theory 1991 Spring;15(1):121-3.

158. Blixrud, op. cit., 49-55.

159. Barker JW. Acquisitions principles and the future of acquisitions: information soup, the soup-hungry, and libraries' five dimensions. Libr Acquis Pract Theory 1993 Spring;17(1):23-32.

160. Gorman, The academic library, op. cit., 9.

2

Monograph Acquisitions

Mark E. Funk

What exactly is a monograph? Commonly known as a book to the general public, a monograph is a one-time publication that is typically complete in one physical volume. Some monographs actually consist of multiple volumes, but the number of volumes is known and specified from the beginning, unlike serials, which have open-ended publication plans. The term "monograph" is also used to denote a research work on a narrowly defined topic, as contrasted to a textbook or popular title. This chapter, however, addresses the issues of acquiring "monographs" in the most general sense of the term. (Chapter 5: Acquisition of Audiovisual and Digital Media deals with the special requirements of acquiring these formats whether issued serially or as one-time publications.)

The acquisition of monographs is one of the oldest functions in libraries. Indeed, until the beginning of scientific journals in the seventeenth century, a collection of monographs was the *sine qua non* of a library. Without the ordering and receipt of books, there was no library, and thus no need for cataloging, reference, or any other services. While other areas in the library reaped the benefit of early automation endeavors, acquisitions procedures, until recently, have remained little changed from those used in the last century. Only since the late 1980s has this basic library function been liberated from the drudgery of routine by the advance of computer technology.

Ironically, as acquisitions departments join the computer age, the decline of the printed book may well be approaching, brought on by the computer itself. While few would argue that the book we know today will disappear completely, most librarians agree that we will depend less on the printed monograph in the future, as electronic methods of information delivery become easier and cheaper. This first edition of *Current Practice in Health Sciences Librarianship* may well be the last to devote an entire chapter to acquiring printed books. However, electronic publications will need to attain three characteristics before they can replace printed monographs: they will need to be commonplace, convenient, and cheap. Until electronic publications achieve these qualities, health science libraries will remain in the business of acquiring printed monographs.

This chapter addresses the complete acquisitions process: from the receipt of the purchase request; to the placing of the order; the receipt of the item; and payment processing. In addition to standard publications from commercial publishers, the chapter covers microforms, government documents, and publications from professional associations. Particular attention has been paid to the various sources available to a library for purchasing monographs. Where applicable, conceptual and procedural differences between large and small health science libraries are discussed. When procedures are described, both manual systems and automated acquisitions systems have been considered.

For the novice in monograph acquisitions, it is easy to be overwhelmed by the number of decisions that need to be made. Should a book be ordered directly from the publisher, or from a book vendor? Which vendor should be used? Should the library prepay with a check, or is a purchase order necessary? How much information about the book should be supplied with the order? Fortunately, the decision-making process can be focused by remembering that the primary goal in acquisitions is to obtain materials needed by the library's users for the best price, and in the most timely and efficient manner. By consistently pursuing this goal, acquisitions decisions will be easier to make.

It is also useful to bear in mind that there are two fundamental aspects to monograph acquisitions, although sometimes it is difficult to separate them. First, there are the internal, library-based processes. These are based on standard information-retrieval methods, record-management techniques, and coordinated interaction with other departments within the library. Experienced library staff, even those new to acquisitions, are familiar with these strategies. Then, there are the external ordering processes: dealing with people and businesses outside the library. Even experienced librarians who are new to acquisitions work may find these external processes daunting. Here, experience and consultation with colleagues are the best teachers. This chapter will address both the internal and external components of the acquisitions process, with an emphasis on the rationale underlying the decision-making process.

The Acquisitions Unit Record

A successful monographs acquisitions operation depends most of all upon a well-structured and well-maintained record keeping system. Such a system should allow library staff to issue purchase orders and other communications to suppliers and to track the status of all outstanding and recently received orders. Whether accomplished through use of an automated system or through a file of printed multipart forms, the goal is to avoid redundant data entry by establishing a single unit record for the order, which is updated as the order moves through the various stages of order entry, claiming (if necessary), receipt, payment, and cataloging.

Computerized Records

Until fairly recently, only the largest health sciences libraries had automated their acquisitions process. In its early years, automation was expensive, complicated, and fraught with dangers of hardware failure, software failure, and even system supplier failure. Automating today is easier, because the available systems are friendlier, more reliable, and less expensive. Boss has summarized the history of automated acquisitions as it has evolved from large mainframes to minicomputers to personal computers [1].

Maintaining a computerized acquisitions system is not a luxury. It has concrete advantages for library users and the library itself. For library users who want information quickly, automated acquisitions can speed up the ordering process. Since almost all automated systems can use bibliographic records downloaded from bibliographic utilities as order records, expensive and time consuming rekeying of data is minimized. Automation is also invaluable because it gives librarians information needed for management decisions. As library materials increase in price, librarians require rapid and accurate analyses of expenditures—where and how the library's money was spent. Even daily reports of expenditures, encumbrances, and funds remaining are easily available through most automated systems. Automated acquisitions can also assist in evaluating book vendor performance, by automatically calculating the average time it takes for orders to be received, or average discounts received. The selection process for an appropriate automated system is a crucial and difficult one; some useful strategies are discussed at the end of this chapter.

Manual Records

Small health science libraries may not need or may not be able to afford an automated acquisitions system. Manual files for tracking the acquisition of library materials have worked for decades, and they can still work today. While the advantages of an automated system are lost, other modern technologies, such as the fax machine, can bring computer-like speed to at least part of the ordering process.

Starting a manual acquisitions system is relatively easy and inexpensive. For a very small departmental library, it can be as simple as typing a list of books wanted, mailing the list to a supplier, and keeping a copy on file. Most libraries, however, require more sophistication than this. A more typical manual system involves typing individual orders onto preprinted multipart order forms. These forms are then separated, with one copy being sent to the supplier, and the rest kept in one or more library files. The copies are arranged to provide different avenues of access, e.g., by title or by budget fund. Carbonless multipart order forms for this purpose are available from most library supply companies, both in standard and customized formats.

Before establishing the format for a printed unit order record, the library's needs for record keeping should be carefully analyzed. These include any statistical reports that might be needed, as well as any requirements by the institution's purchasing or accounting departments. Because the order form, or a copy of it, may be the only record created for an item, there should be space on the form for internal library information. This internal information might include a sequential purchase order number, the account to be charged, both the date ordered and date received, the final cost of the item, and the location where the item is to be placed. A basic preprinted book purchase order form might look like the one in Figure 2-1.

Although a library can use the copies of an order form in any way that provides functionality, possible uses include

- Copy to send to book supplier. This is usually the top copy, with the clearest type. Some libraries have special order instructions preprinted on the back of this copy, such as invoicing and shipping instructions.

- Library copy for on-order file.

- Copy to file in card catalog or shelf list. This is usually the bottom copy of the forms, on card or ledger stock, with a prepunched hole for easy filing.

<table>
<tr><td colspan="2" align="center">Book Purchase Order</td></tr>
<tr><td colspan="2">Author:
Title:

Place: Publisher:
Edition or series: Volumes: Year:
ISBN: Price: No. of copies:
Special Instructions:</td></tr>
<tr><td>Order Number:</td><td>Date Ordered:</td></tr>
<tr><td>Location:</td><td>Date Received:</td></tr>
<tr><td>Account:</td><td>Actual Cost:</td></tr>
<tr><td>From: Acquisitions Dept.
      Health Sciences Library
      123 Main St.
      Anytown, USA</td><td>To:</td></tr>
</table>

Figure 2-1: A Basic Book Purchase Order Form

- Library copy for fund file, to permit convenient production of fiscal reports.

- Library copy filed by order date, to expedite claiming overdue items.

Most libraries find it easiest to arrange their on-order file by title instead of by author or by purchase order number [2]. As anyone who has done cataloging will attest, assigning authorship is sometimes a complex and judgmental process, particularly for corporate entries. Title filing can be done without recourse to cataloging rules. Also, since the suppliers' order reports and invoices often list only titles, matching is easier with a title arrangement.

The primary problems with a manual acquisitions system are the hidden personnel expenses of maintaining it and the limited options for retrieving and summarizing subsets of records (e.g., by subject, fund, or order status). Correcting typing errors on multipart forms is difficult at best, and often impossible. Separating and filing the different parts is very labor intensive and prone to errors. Retrieving information from manual files or summarizing it for fiscal and statistical reports can be difficult and time consuming.

When budgeting for a manual acquisitions system, the personnel time required to maintain it should not be underestimated.

The Acquisition Process

To understand the ordering process, it is crucial to understand the various methods of procurement available. The two basic modes of procurement are firm orders, i.e., orders sent to either publishers or vendors for specific items, and approval plans, i.e., arrangements by which books are received automatically upon publication, based on an established profile of library interests.

Firm Orders

When a specific book is required by the library, a firm order is sent to the appropriate supplier, generally either the publisher or a wholesale book vendor for titles that are still in-print. Although larger libraries tend to favor the use of book vendors, there are sometimes compelling reasons to order directly from the publisher. Reasons for ordering a book directly from the publisher include the following:

- For some publishers, this is the only way to acquire their publications, because they do not accept orders through book vendors.

- It is sometimes quicker to receive a book directly from a publisher, especially if the book is on their backlist (i.e., not a recently published title).

- Ordering from a publisher keeps the library on the publisher's mailing list for catalogs and new book announcements.

A book vendor (also called a book jobber) is a wholesaler that supplies books to libraries and bookstores. Book vendors derive a profit because, in buying in bulk from publishers, they receive a discount off the list price. In many cases, the vendor can pass on some of that discount to the library. The difference between the discount that vendors receive and the discount they pass on to libraries is what pays the vendors' expenses and contributes to their profits. The advantages to using a vendor instead of a publisher include the following:

- For many publishers' titles, the library receives a discount off the list price.

- Consolidation of a large batch of orders to a vendor streamlines the entire acquisitions process — one order out, one shipment in, and one invoice to process.

- Prepayment is usually not required. This means the order can be processed by the vendor as soon as it is received. There is no delay in waiting for the library's institution to write a check, and no delay for the publisher waiting for a check to clear.

- Many vendors do not charge for postage or handling.

- Most vendors provide follow-up reports on orders, informing the library of delays or other problems.

A fuller discussion on deciding where to send firm orders is to be found later in this chapter in the section "Sources of Materials."

Approval Plans

Although an approval plan is primarily a collection development tool, many aspects are managed by the acquisitions department. An approval plan, as noted above, involves the automatic receipt of books, usually from a commercial book vendor, that have matched a library's collecting needs as defined by an approval "profile." These books are sent to the library "on approval." Books that are not wanted by the library are returned. Books that are "approved" by the library are kept and paid for. Some publishers offer similar approval plans restricted to their own publications.

A useful adjunct to an approval plan is a slips service. With a slips service, the library does not automatically receive the books that meet specified profile requirements. Instead, the vendor sends preprinted order slips containing full bibliographic information on these books. The library's book selectors choose which items they wish to see on approval, and return the slips to the vendor. The selected items appear in a subsequent approval shipment, where they are treated like all other approval books.

Preorder Processes

No matter where the request to purchase a book originates (library user or library selector), it is important to verify basic items of information before an order can be sent out. First, it must be determined that the item is not already in the library or on order. Second, a full and accurate bibliographic description of the item must be obtained. This two-part process is called preorder searching or preorder verification. It is done to prevent the library from ordering something that it has already ordered or received, and to verify that the item actually exists by confirming its bibliographic description in an authoritative source.

Elimination of Duplicate Orders

In most cases, a check of both the public catalog and the file of titles on order is enough to identify duplicate orders. One of the advantages of a computerized integrated library system (ILS) that displays on-order records in the public catalog is that only a single search is required to discover duplicate orders.

Even in this seemingly simple process, however, experience plays an important role, since identifying a duplicate can sometimes be problematic. Occasionally publishers produce a monograph consisting of material that originally appeared as a journal issue or journal supplement, but neglect to mention this information in their advertising. Other publishers may reprint a government publication under a new title, failing to mention the original title, which may already be in the library's collection. Only with experience, a high degree of suspicion, and by checking multiple access points can these culprits be caught before ordering.

If the request to purchase an item already owned by the library was made by a library user, the library should notify the requester that the item is already in the collection. If the requested item is already on order, the library may want to add the requester's name to the original order, so that he or she can be notified when it becomes available.

Many libraries, as part of the preorder searching process, annotate the purchase request to show the call number of any previous or related editions already in the collection. This information is passed on for later use in the cataloging process.

Bibliographic Verification

There must be sufficient, accurate information on the order form sent to the supplier so that the one unique item can be identified and not confused with any other item. When an order is based on a listing in a recent publisher catalog or on an advertising brochure (often referred to as a "blurb"), the library may need to look no further for reliable bibliographic and ordering information. However, orders that are based on recommendations from library users or on brief entries in subject bibliographies typically require further research to validate and complete the bibliographic identification. This is especially true if no International Standard Book Number (ISBN) has been provided, since the ISBN is the single most reliable way of identifying a published work unambiguously. Other elements of item identification that may need to be checked for accuracy include author, title, edition, publisher, year of publication, series, price, and format (hardcover or paperback).

Most libraries have a purchase request form that indicates the items of bibliographic identification required from the selector or the library user, but it cannot be assumed that the form will be filled out completely or accurately. For this reason, bibliographic verification should not be considered a low-skill activity, assigned to inexperienced staff members. While a majority of preorder searches may require reference to only one or two sources of verification, some requests will require extensive searching. This is particularly true for books issued by small specialty publishers, private presses, and many non-U.S. publishers.

Verification Tools

In the past, acquisitions departments often maintained a large arsenal of expensive and voluminous bibliographic tools they could use to verify book orders. This was particularly true in libraries that attempted to create comprehensive collections. For better or worse, those days are gone. A combination of shrinking budgets and an ever-shortening window of in-print availability has decreased the need for maintaining more than a few verification tools. In addition, easy access to a wide variety of electronic databases has replaced many of the bulky printed tools.

Publishers' Catalogs

Most health science libraries maintain a file of publishers' catalogs for both collection development and acquisitions reference. One might expect that a publisher's catalog would have accurate information and could be used as a definitive source. In most cases, catalog information is indeed accurate. However, publishers' information occasionally contains incorrect ISBNs, the wrong authors or misspelled authors' names, and even incorrect titles, especially for items that have been announced in advance of their actual publication. Current prices are often higher than the prices listed in the catalog, and projected dates of publications can be months or even years too optimistic.

Many health science publishers are attentive to sending the latest version of their catalogs to libraries. However, other publishers automatically send catalogs only to customers who order directly from them. Libraries that order from vendors often miss receiving these catalogs, and must request them in writing. It is especially useful to have up-to-date catalogs and price lists for publishers that require prepayment. Since files of publishers' catalogs grow quickly, an annual weeding of the file helps to maintain a manageable size and to identify missing or out-of-date catalogs. A growing number of publishers are now making their catalogs available on the Internet. A comprehensive, regularly updated list of these publishers can be found on the World Wide Web at the AcqWeb home page (http://www.library.vanderbilt.edu/law/acqs/acqs.html).

Books in Print and Related Tools

Books in Print (BIP), published by R.R. Bowker, is an annual listing of in-print books distributed in the United States. Full order information is usually included for every entry. The basic *BIP* set lists books by both title and author, and includes addresses and phone numbers of U.S. publishers and distributors. A separate *Subject Guide to Books in Print* is also available. *BIP* is outdated the day after it is published, so its publisher has created accessory publications to update it. *Books in Print Supplement* is published six months after the annual edition, and a bimonthly publication called *Forthcoming Books* lists both recently published and newly announced books. A version of *BIP* is also available on CD-ROM, called *BIP Plus*. Some automated acquisitions systems can interface with *BIP Plus*, allowing both verification and downloading of the bibliographic information into the library's acquisitions system. A specialized version of *BIP* is *Medical and Health Care Books and Serials in Print*. This annual publication is a subset of *BIP* that lists only books and serials on the subjects of medicine, psychiatry, dentistry, nursing, and allied health. Small health sciences libraries may find that this last tool will fill most of their needs.

Larger libraries that purchase heavily from non-U.S. publishers may require additional sources. *International Books in Print* lists English language titles published in Canada, continental Europe, Latin America, Oceania, Africa, Asia, and the Republic of Ireland. *Whitaker's Books in Print* (formerly titled *British Books in Print*) covers books published and distributed in the United Kingdom.

Vendors' Lists and Databases

Most book vendors specializing in health sciences literature send lists of recent publications to their customers, usually arranged in subject order. If selections for purchase have been made from these lists, they can almost always be considered verified. Many vendors maintain either a microfiche listing or online database of books they have in stock. For their own customers, vendors usually allow free online access to this database, which can be used for verification purposes as well as to order items. Many of the vendors' lists and databases also include information as to when books are going out-of-print, and when new editions are due to be published.

Bibliographic Networks

Most academic libraries use one of the major bibliographic utilities such as OCLC or RLIN for cataloging purposes, but they can be used for verification purposes as well. Their strength lies in the fact that the databases are tremendous in size, improving the likelihood of success in finding a particular record. In addition, most automated acquisitions systems can accommodate online downloading of OCLC or RLIN records, thus eliminating the rekeying of order records. However, most of these records do not include a price, and many of the records of recent publications are Cataloging-in-Publication (CIP) copy, which can be incomplete or inaccurate. Acquisitions personnel need to be trained to search these utilities, unless the cataloging department is performing the verification process.

National Library of Medicine's CATLINE

Smaller health science libraries that may not have access to OCLC or RLIN can also use the National Library of Medicine's CATLINE database to verify titles. CATLINE contains bibliographic records for printed monographs and serials in biomedicine. Since NLM participates in the CIP program with the Library of Congress, CATLINE contains thousands of records of just published or soon-to-be-published books, which are usually what libraries want to order. A special print command (PRT AC) prints the fields necessary for acquisitions purposes. CATLINE records include prices of items if they were available at the time of cataloging, but this field is not updated when prices change. Prices are in U.S. dollars only.

Assigning Internal Ordering Information

While the standard bibliographic elements are all that are necessary to specify an order, most libraries add additional elements to the order record as part of the acquisition process. These elements provide necessary or useful pieces of information for payment, processing, and statistics.

Purchase Order Number

Unless a library is so small that it orders only a very limited number of items, it typically assigns an individual purchase order (P.O.) number to each item ordered. Many publishers require such a P.O. number for institutional purchases. From the library's perspective, this number also makes it much easier to match up the items, vendor reports, and invoices when they are received. Sequential numbers also allow easy calculation of the number of orders sent out in any time period. Procedures for assigning these numbers vary. If all orders must go through an institutional purchasing department before they are sent out, that department may assign the number, which is then reported to the library. Most automated acquisitions systems can automatically assign a new number to each item entered into the system. Libraries using manual systems may either obtain purchase order forms with sequential numbers preprinted on them; use a sequential numbering stamper; or assign sequential numbers manually.

Budget Account

If a library uses more than one budget account to purchase its materials, it is essential that the correct account name or code be added to the order record. Frequently, these accounts are identified officially by a long string of alphanumeric characters. If at all possible, it is advisable to use a simpler code name for these different accounts for internal library processing, to reduce the inevitable keyboarding errors.

Subject Code

The acquisitions department may want to assign a general subject heading or code to each order. For both collection development and budget preparation, a breakdown of annual purchases by subjects can be useful. Many automated systems allow the library to maintain a list of controlled subject terms that can be assigned to orders.

Type of Order

Most purchases in acquisitions are for titles new to the collection, but orders for additional copies or replacement of lost or damaged volumes are not uncommon. For collection development or budget preparation purposes, a library may wish to know how much was spent on new items, replacement items, and additional copies.

Name of Requester

If items being ordered have been specifically requested or recommended for purchase by library users, those requesters may wish to be notified after the item has been processed and ready for use. If so, the requester's name should be added to the order record. The requester's address and phone number may also be useful.

Information for Cataloging

Acquisitions and cataloging departments commonly work closely together. The original purchase request often contains information that cataloging requires, and the preorder verification process can also add additional information. It is important that this information be passed on to the cataloging department, so that this information doesn't need to be located a second time. Data potentially useful for cataloging include

- Previous editions of the item in the collection.

- Other copies of the item in the collection.

- Whether item is a replacement or added copy.

- Shelving location of item (e.g., general stacks, Reserve, Reference).

- Circulation restrictions of the item.

- Name of requester to be notified.

- Special funding source or name of donor (often used for special bookplates).

Most automated acquisitions systems have fields where this information can be entered into the order record. After the book has been received, some systems produce a special acquisitions/cataloging processing slip containing bibliographic information and all of the added processing data. This slip is then placed in the book before it goes to cataloging. Many libraries without this capability have created their own acquisitions/cataloging form, which acquisitions personnel fill out during the verification process and pass on to cataloging along with the item.

Order Transmission

Mail Ordering

Libraries generally send out book orders on a regular schedule. Small libraries that order few books may send an order out as soon as it has been completed. However, large libraries that order many books may find it advantageous to batch the mailing of their orders to consolidate processing time and reduce mailing costs. Of course, orders needed quickly should be printed or typed right away, and sent as soon as possible. Given the minimum delay of three to five days for mail delivery of orders to book suppliers, faster options should be considered for "rush" orders.

A convenient feature for both automated and manual acquisitions is a printed order form on which the supplier's address can be seen in a window envelope. This feature eliminates the need for typing of addresses on each envelope.

Telephone Ordering

Most vendors have toll-free numbers that can be used to order books. The telephone is fast and convenient, and no extra equipment is necessary.

However, there are more chances for transcription errors on both the library and vendor side, and it is cumbersome to order more than a few books this way. This option should be reserved for single "rush" orders. To avoid problems, all phone orders should be fully documented for future reference (date, time, and name of the person who took the order). Although many publishers also have toll-free order numbers, they typically require pre-payment with a credit card, a mode of payment which can not be accommodated in most institutions.

Electronic Ordering

EDI: X12 and EDIFACT Standards

While many libraries, vendors, and publishers have used automated ordering systems for years, getting the order from the library to the supplier has still depended largely on the postal system. With the proliferation of electronic communication options, however, many businesses have seen the advantages of sending orders directly from their computer to their supplier's computer. In the early years of this electronic data interchange (EDI), there were no standards, and businesses had to customize their software to accommodate the different EDI codes used by their vendors and customers. While standards have developed over the years, there are currently competing standards, resulting in some confusion.

- X12 standards: created by the American National Standards Institute's Accredited Standards Committee X12 (ANSI ASC X12) in 1979. These are the EDI standards now used most commonly in the United States.

- EDIFACT standards: created by the United Nations Economic Commission for Europe. EDIFACT (EDI for Administration, Commerce, and Transport), approved by the International Organization for Standardization in 1987, has different standards from X12.

Fortunately, the members of ANSI ASC X12 have voted to adopt the EDIFACT standards beginning in 1997, thus creating a single, world-wide standard [3]. When fully implemented, EDI standards will allow a library to send an electronic book order to any participating vendor or publisher. The order will include the necessary bibliographic information as well as the shipping address. The supplier's computer will respond by acknowledging the order and indicating when the book will be shipped. Claims from the library for outstanding orders and claim responses will also be processed electronically, with no human intervention.

There is a high demand in the marketplace for the implementation of EDI standards by book vendors and in automated library systems. While future automated systems will be designed with EDI standards built into them, libraries with existing systems may have to wait until the system's designers develop EDI translator programs.

Vendor Systems

Most book vendors have already automated their internal systems for book ordering, invoicing, and inventory. As more and more libraries purchased microcomputers and modems in the 1980s, it wasn't very difficult for these vendors to provide access to their internal computer files for their customers. Using either proprietary software (usually provided free by the vendor) or a simple telecommunications program, a library can dial into its vendor's system, browse the inventory, enter new orders, and inquire about outstanding orders.

Some vendors allow their online records to be downloaded to the library's computerized acquisitions system, saving the rekeying of this data. In what may be a trend, a few vendors are also enriching their bibliographic records by adding the tables of contents of individual books, which not only can be searched, but also downloaded and added to the cataloging record. For libraries using manual systems, most vendors offering dial-in service can, at the library's option, mail confirmation of orders on multipart forms. This procedure is a relatively inexpensive and easy way to speed the ordering process. If a library uses more than one book vendor, however, acquisitions personnel need to learn each vendor's system.

Fax and E-mail Ordering

Even small, nonautomated libraries can speed their orders electronically by using a fax machine or electronic mail (e-mail). Fax requires an extra piece of equipment, but most libraries now have fax machines, or access to one. While most fax phone numbers are not toll-free, it takes little time to send even several pages of orders. An additional advantage is that an accurate record of the library's orders is produced at the other end, which means fewer chances for errors.

In response to customer demand, many book vendors have also set up Internet e-mail accounts. Libraries can use this simple and fast method of sending orders to a vendor. Depending on how a library accesses e-mail, there may be telecommunication charges with this method. However, like fax, it is fast, relatively inexpensive, and an accurate record of orders is produced at the other end. E-mail also eliminates the nuisance of busy signals while trying to fax an order. In both fax and e-mail ordering, a library may want to request a confirmation that the order has been received.

Receiving Materials

Checking for Accuracy and Completeness

When receiving materials ordered, the boxes must be unpacked, the books sorted, and the items then matched to the original order and to the invoice or packing slip. The receiver must answer several important questions: Did all of the items listed on the packing skip or invoice arrive? Do the items correctly match the orders? For each item, is the author, title, edition, format, price, and number of copies correct? Each book should be examined briefly and checked for blank or damaged pages or broken bindings. Before the boxes are discarded, the packing material should be examined, to make sure that no books or invoices have been left inside.

Depending on the vendor or the library's preferences, invoices for monographs may be included with the shipped items, or sent separately. The actual invoiced cost of each item should be checked against the order record. Small differences in price are usually due to either a greater or lesser discount than anticipated, and shipping and handling charges may have been added. Infrequently, large differences between the ordered price and the actual price may be discovered. Some of these discrepancies are due to library or vendor errors, but occasionally a publisher drastically increases the price of a title soon after it has been published. Large price discrepancies should be investigated, and possibly discussed with the selector before an invoice is approved for payment. To prevent such surprises, some libraries ask their vendors to notify them before shipping if the actual price of a book will be more than a specified amount over the ordered price.

When an item has been received, its status must be changed in the on-order file. In an automated system, it is easy to call up the order, verify it against the book in hand, and then change the status of the item to indicate it has been received. In a manual system, the order forms need to be pulled from the on-order file, matched against the books, annotated with the date received, and then refiled into the received file.

Approving and Posting Payment

If the invoice correctly reflects the items received, it may be approved for payment. Few libraries actually make payments by producing the checks themselves. In most cases, an internal document called a payment voucher is filled out, which authorizes the accounts payable department of the institution to issue a check to the supplier. The payment voucher is usually a sequentially numbered multipart form, but electronic forms are becoming common as more accounting departments become automated. Information required on the payment voucher varies between institutions, but at a minimum the voucher must clearly state the name and address of the supplier, as well as the invoice number and its date, the amount to be paid, and the account(s) to be used. Some institutions require a brief description of the purchased item(s), and almost all institutions require an authorized signature on the voucher [4]. Many institutions require that the supplier's federal employer identification number (FEIN) be included as well, if it is not shown on the invoice. The original invoice accompanies the voucher to the institution's accounts payable department. Multiple copies of the invoice may be required, and most book vendors can customize their invoices to meet local requirements. One copy of both the voucher and the invoice is normally retained by the library.

Payment approvals should be processed with a minimum of delay. After processing by acquisitions staff, payment vouchers may go through several different departments before a check is issued. This lack of direct control over payment means that checks occasionally get delayed or misrouted. Since the supplier has sent the books in good faith, the library should make every effort to pay the supplier promptly.

Invoice Adjustments

For shipments of a single book arriving with a single invoice, invoice approval is uncomplicated. However, when a large shipment arrives, there are more chances of problems with the invoice or the shipment: an incorrect book may have been sent, a book may have been damaged during transit, or the invoice may be incorrect. Procedures should be worked out with both the vendor and the institution's accounting department for the smooth handling of these common problems. Obviously, if these problems are occurring regularly, the vendor needs to be notified of the library's concern. Vendors and publishers vary on how they handle the invoices for partial shipments or items being returned. The institution's accounting department may also have requirements for invoice adjustments. Four methods are commonly used by libraries [5]:

Credit memo

The supplier issues the library a credit memo that can be deducted against the current invoice, if the library has not yet paid. If the library has already paid the invoice, the credit memo can be deducted from a later invoice.

Striking from the invoice

The library amends the invoice by lining out the erroneous or returned item, and subtracting its amount from the total.

Requesting a new, corrected invoice

This method usually delays payment but may be preferred by the parent institution.

Returning the invoice with the item

This option can be used only if the invoice has a single item on it.

Posting Payment

The final operation of the receiving process is to post, or record, the payment for each item in the individual order record. After posting, each completed acquisitions record will have not only all of the original order information and the date the item was received, it will also have the invoice number and its date, the amount paid, the payment voucher number (if one is used), and the date the payment was processed. In a manual filing system, this information can be recorded on the purchase order copy that was pulled from the on-order file. If a manual ledger for tracking expenditures is being maintained, payment is posted to it. Once payment is posted, the purchase order can be placed in the completed orders file. Automated acquisitions systems allow rapid posting by calling up the order record and adding the posting information to it. The amount encumbered for each item is automatically zeroed out, and the expenditure is deducted from the account charged.

Precataloging Processing

If a library uses an acquisitions/cataloging processing form, this form is inserted into the book before it is sent on to cataloging. Automated systems that produce processing forms may allow batch printing of the forms for books received that day, or can print out forms for each book as soon as its status changes from "on-order" to "received."

Some acquisitions departments also record the price, vendor, date received, and the account charged in an inconspicuous place in each book. Other acquisitions departments may be responsible for adding property stamps, book plates, security strips, or sending paperbacks for binding.

Receiving Approval Plan Shipments

Receiving materials in an approval shipment requires slightly different procedures than those for firm orders, since these items arrive with no preorder searching or records preceding them. Most libraries follow procedures similar to the following for receiving approval plans.

- Verify the package contents against the packing list or invoice.

- Check the approval items against the catalog and on-order file to detect duplicates.

- If previous editions of a book exist, check as to whether the library owns any. This information is helpful to selectors and catalogers.

- Assign purchase order number, budget account, subject code, and type of order.

Some libraries enter all of the approval items into their acquisitions system, and then indicate which items were returned by selectors. Other libraries enter into the system only the items retained by selectors.

Returns

The staff member responsible for receiving monograph orders must understand the importance of verifying their accuracy and completeness. In an ideal world, every order received would be completely accurate and in perfect condition. In the real world, vendors and publishers sometimes send the wrong item, or send two copies of a book when only one was ordered. Occasionally, a book may be defective or damaged during transit. Problem books like these must be returned.

Most vendors allow the library to send returns back to them, with a note explaining the problem. The return note should identify both the library and the account. Prior authorization for returns is normally not required. Before returning items directly to publishers, however, their customer service department should be contacted to get return instructions if these are not included on the invoice or packing slip. Many publishers require returned items to be sent to a special address. Some publishers require returns to be identified with a special shipping label which they supply, and some may require postal insurance or United Parcel Service shipping. In all cases, it is wise to mail returns by some form of traceable mail, to protect the library in cases of dispute.

Claims

Although most monograph orders arrive from the publisher or vendor within a reasonable time, there are occasional orders that remain outstanding too long. When this happens, the library needs to enter a claim for these books. Knowing when to claim an item is crucial in maintaining both prompt delivery and good vendor relations. Claiming too soon after an order is sent out, or too soon between follow-up claims, causes more work for both the library and the vendor. The Bookdealer–Library Relations Committee of the American Library Association has established reasonable delivery dates for in-print monographs [6]. Claims may be made when these waiting periods have been exceeded:

- U.S. commercial publications should be supplied within 90 days.

- U.S. noncommercial publications should be supplied within 120 days.

- Foreign commercial publications should be supplied within 180 days.

- Follow-up claims can be placed 30 days after previous claims for U.S. publications.

These claiming schedules are intended as guidelines. The library's vendor or colleagues at other libraries may have different suggestions for reasonable claiming schedules.

For manual on-order files maintained in title order, the entire file must be examined for possible claims. If the library also maintains an extra copy of the order form filed by order date, it is relatively easy to determine which items need claiming. An automated system should allow the library to determine its own claiming schedule, and automatically produce claims at proper intervals. In either case, the library should update the order record with the date and number of the latest claim.

Claim Forms

A claim is usually a simple form sent to the order supplier, which identifies an order and its order date, indicates that it hasn't been received, and requests the supplier to update the status of the order. Claim forms are sometimes provided by the book vendor the library uses. If not, they may be ordered from library supply companies, or custom-printed by a printing company. Some libraries photocopy the order forms and attach them to a claim letter. Automated acquisitions systems can produce claim forms on demand. A typical claim form may look like Figure 2-2.

If a second or third claim is necessary, the number of the claim should be noted on the form. Some libraries leave a space on the claim form for the supplier's reply, other libraries rely on the supplier's own claim response reports.

<table>
<tr><td colspan="2" align="center">Claim Notice
This Is Not An Order</td></tr>
<tr><td>From: Acquisitions Dept.
      Health Sciences Library
      123 Main St.
      Anytown, USA</td><td>To:</td></tr>
<tr><td colspan="2">Claim Number: Date:
The following order is overdue. Please update its order status.</td></tr>
<tr><td colspan="2">Author: Title:

Publisher: Edition: Year:
ISBN: Price: No. of copies:
Order number: Order Date:</td></tr>
</table>

Figure 2-2: A Typical Claim Form

Electronic Claiming

When the EDI electronic order standards are in place, many automated acquisitions systems will be able to send claims to suppliers electronically. In turn, the suppliers' computers will respond electronically to the claims, updating the library's order record in the process. Until then, claims may be speeded to vendors through older electronic technology such as fax and e-mail.

Claim Reports and Order Status Updates

In addition to responding to specific claims, vendors send out periodic reports indicating the status of all outstanding orders. For example, a book may have been delayed in publication, or the vendor may have received the wrong book from the publisher, and had to reorder. This information should be entered into the order records so that the library doesn't claim a book just after it has been reported as delayed. A good automated system should allow entry of a predicted delivery date based on a vendor report, and then automatically skip claiming an item until this date has passed.

Most vendors and publishers use standard abbreviations or phrases for their claims responses and status reports. The following are commonly seen:

NYR (Not yet received)

The vendor has placed the order with the publisher, and it is considered an active order.

OS (Out-of-stock)

This is usually a response from a vendor that warehouses books. No copies are at the vendor, but an order has been placed with the publisher.

OSI (Out-of-stock indefinitely)

Publisher out-of-stock. While there is a slight chance of a future reprint, this happens very rarely. In effect, this is a cancellation.

NYP (Not yet published)

If known, most vendors report the expected date of publication.

Claiming

The order is active, and the vendor is claiming from the publisher.

OP (Out-of-print)

The order is canceled. Many publishers report "OP" to a vendor when supplies are low. Occasionally it is possible to order a copy directly from the publisher. However, an "OP" report from a publisher is definitive.

NOP (Not our publication)

The publisher has reported to the vendor that the ordered title is not theirs. The vendor has canceled the order. The item must be reverified and reordered.

Cannot supply

The vendor is unable to supply this item. The order has been canceled, and must be reordered from another source.

Cancellations

Cancellations of on-order items are either supplier initiated or library initiated. Most cancellations from vendors and publishers occur because the item is out-of-print or cannot otherwise be supplied.

Rarely, a library may want to cancel an order because it was ordered in error, or a copy was received as a gift after the order was created. This type of cancellation should be infrequent, because an order is a promise to purchase and pay, and a cancellation may represent financial loss to the vendor. The library and the vendor should both have a clear understanding of when these cancellations are allowable.

Many libraries cancel an order if it has been outstanding for too long, for example, over one year, with no predicted delivery date. Other libraries, because of institutional requirements, may have to cancel all outstanding orders at the end of a fiscal year. Again, both the library and the vendor should understand these procedures when they start doing business.

Cancellation forms, like claim forms, should contain enough information for the supplier to identify the item being canceled. They should contain the date, and a clear notice that it represents a cancellation. Many libraries also include the reason for cancellation on the form.

Sources of Materials

In deciding which supplier to use for a given book, it is useful to remember the basic goal of acquisitions: obtaining materials for the best price and in the most timely and efficient manner. While some items can only be ordered directly from the publisher, most monographs can be ordered through a variety of sources. The following points should be considered:

- Pricing. Can the supplier provide the item at a discount?

- Speed. How soon can delivery be expected from the supplier?

- Accuracy. Does the supplier have a good track record of accuracy?

- Ease of ordering and payment. How easy is it to process orders and payments for this supplier?

Book Vendors

Selecting a Book Vendor

There are many book vendors eager for the library's business, and, in most cases, vendors take the initiative in making themselves known to potential library customers. Most vendors that specialize in the health science field exhibit at the annual meeting of the Medical Library Association (MLA), and many of them also exhibit at the regional meetings of MLA chapters. These meetings are good places to collect information on vendors' services—both from the vendors and from colleagues. A new acquisitions librarian should not be reticent about asking other librarians what vendors they use and what they think of them. Most of them will be glad to offer their opinions. However, it is wise to get a broad range of opinion, since what works (or doesn't work) for one library may not apply to another library. Also, service from the larger vendors may depend upon the quality of the regional office or warehouse serving the area.

Although it is generally true that the commercial library supply industry is volatile at best (with takeovers and business failures a common feature), the quartet of major U.S. biomedical book vendors has remained remarkably stable over the years: Majors Scientific Books (Dallas, TX), Login Brothers Book Company (Chicago, IL), Matthews Medical Books (Maryland Heights, MO), and Rittenhouse Books Distributors (King of Prussia, PA). There was a time when these companies operated almost entirely on the basis of mutually exclusive geographic regions, however they now promote their services on a nationwide basis. Other well-established book vendors that can provide a broad range of scientific and other academic titles include Baker & Taylor and Blackwell North America. Advertisements in *Library Journal* and similar publications can provide additional prospects.

After potential book vendors have been identified, how does the acquisitions librarian decide which one to use? In some cases, the librarian may not have a choice. Some state, federal, or city libraries may be required to use a book vendor selected by the parent institution. Other libraries, because of local requirements, may be required to award a vendor contract through a bidding process. Unfortunately, the bidding process often emphasizes discount over service, and awarding a contract to the lowest bidder may ultimately cause a deterioration in timely delivery of ordered books. If bids are required, it is important to write a clear and detailed Request For Proposal (RFP) to send to potential vendors, and then to monitor the performance of the selected vendor(s) [7-8].

If the choice of book vendor is up to the librarian, the process should be treated as seriously as hiring an assistant. First, the candidates should be narrowed down to those who would appear to best match the library's needs. Then, an appointment can be set up with each qualified vendor for an interview in the library. During the vendors' presentations, it is important to include all of the acquisitions staff who would be communicating with the vendor. As in a job interview, many librarians find it useful to have a set of questions to ask each vendor.

Potential questions for book vendors might include

- What are the added services that the vendor can offer? (Can card sets be supplied with the books? Can the vendor start an out-of-print search for titles reported as out-of-print?)

- Are "rush" orders treated as such?

- Does the vendor assign a single customer service representative to an account to guarantee continuity of service?

- Does the vendor maintain a warehouse of books, or are most orders passed on to publishers? How many titles are usually available for immediate shipment?

- Which publishers does the vendor routinely handle, and what are the normal discounts offered for each?

- Can the vendor supply a list of publishers that it will not handle?

- How often are status reports produced?

- What other management reports are available?

- Are telephone and fax orders acceptable?

- Does the vendor have an online system that can receive orders electronically from the library's automated system?

- Is the vendor's inventory searchable online, so that availability can be immediately known?

- Is there flexibility in how invoices are produced? (Can they be listed by purchase order number, by account, and alphabetically by author or title?)

- Who are some current customers that could be contacted?

Like job applicants, vendors are trying to sell themselves to the library. The librarian must not succumb to sales pressure and must not make a premature decision. A decision should be made only after all the qualified vendors have been met, and after they have been discussed with the acquisitions staff. If it is difficult to decide between two vendors, both can be tried simultaneously and evaluated after six months. However, if a library tests two vendors simultaneously, it should be careful to send both vendors a similar mix of orders (domestic publishers, foreign publishers, current imprints, and older imprints), so they can be compared fairly.

Many small health science libraries find that using the services of a single, biomedical book vendor satisfies all of their needs. Larger libraries, and those that occasionally require nonhealth science books, often use multiple book vendors. There are, for example, book vendors that specialize in British books, university press books, or continental European books. In some cases, specialty vendors can supply these books faster and sometimes cheaper than biomedical vendors. The decision to use one or more book vendors depends on the particular acquisitions needs of each library.

After a decision has been made on which vendor to use, it is a good practice to telephone or write the other vendors who also made a presentation. These presentations cost the vendors time and money, and courtesy requires that they be notified that they were not selected. Most vendors understand that this decision is difficult and that situations may change in the future. For the library, there are obvious benefits to maintaining cordial relationships with potential as well as actual business partners.

Setting Up a Firm Order Account

A newly chosen vendor requires specific information about the particular needs of the library and the parent institution. The following information is easy to obtain, and sharing it with the new vendor may prevent misunderstandings and delays later on.

- Specific invoicing and payment requirements. A copy of these requirements can usually be obtained from the institution's purchasing or accounts payable departments.

- A copy of the order form currently used by the library.

- Special packing or addressing requirements (e.g., room number, department name.)

- A copy of any tax-exempt certificate indicating the library is not to be charged sales tax.

- The day-to-day contact person at the library, including phone number, fax number, and e-mail address.

Conversely, the library should obtain mailing and contact information from the vendor. Most vendors can supply a handbook of information useful in expediting library-vendor communication.

Some libraries find it useful to set up more than one account with a book vendor. Multiple accounts can sometimes simplify fund accounting in larger libraries, where funding often comes from several sources. Even smaller libraries may find multiple accounts more convenient, especially if funding is tied to specific subjects. If multiple accounts are used with vendors, it is important that the correct account number be included on every order that the library sends.

Setting Up an Approval Plan

In setting up an approval plan, book selectors usually establish the profile. Depending on the vendor and the type of plan, the profile may be a set of subjects matching the collecting needs of the library, a set of publishers whose output matches the library's needs, or a combination of the two. Often, nonsubject modifiers are used to further refine the profile. For example, the profile may specify that books over a certain price not be included, or books of a certain format not be included, such as pocket-size books, reprints, or proceedings of meetings. A successful approval plan offers many advantages for collection development.

For acquisitions purposes, an approval plan offers the advantage of speed (books are received soon after they are published), a regular discount, no orders to send out, and fewer invoices to process. Approval plans also eliminate the verification process, since the actual book is in hand. The only searching required is in the public catalog and on-order file, to detect possible duplicates.

The staff member responsible for book selection usually initiates the decision to start an approval plan, but acquisitions staff should be involved in choosing the vendor. Most of the large book vendors offer approval plans. Choosing which plan is best for a particular library will depend on several factors, although of prime importance is the vendor's coverage of the health science literature. Some vendors are better at covering foreign publishers, some are better with university presses, and others are better with clinical health science titles. Discount is one factor to consider but shouldn't be the only one. For selectors, the vendor's coverage and ability to follow the approval plan profile are of utmost importance. For acquisitions, additional factors to consider include

- Speed with which new titles are made available after publication.

- Ease of handling the approval invoices, returns, and credits.

- Frequency and size of approval shipments.

- Shipping charges, including charges for return of rejected volumes.

- Type and usefulness of the vendor's approval plan management reports.

Managing the Approval Plan

As previously mentioned, approval plans offer advantages in the acquisitions process as well as in collection development. But unlike firm orders, on which collection development staff and acquisitions staff can work somewhat independently, an approval plan requires continuous cooperation between the two departments, to maximize its effectiveness.

Of primary concern to acquisitions is the need to avoid sending out a firm order for a book only to have it arrive by way of the approval plan. When this happens, either the firm order must be canceled, or the approval book returned. To prevent inadvertent duplication, acquisitions staff must have a clear understanding of the approval plan profile. If the profile is simple, such as all publications from a list of specified publishers, it is easy to intercept a purchase request for a book from a profiled publisher. However, if the profile consists of subject areas alone or a combination of subjects and publishers, the situation is not so clear cut. Here, the vendor's approval plan selector must interpret the approval plan in deciding whether or not to send each book. It may therefore be unclear to acquisitions staff whether a requested title can safely be anticipated through the approval plan or instead needs to be firm ordered.

There are basically two ways to handle this "order or wait" dilemma. One method is to place purchase requests that might show up on approval into a temporary holding file. Each request should be dated. This file is then checked at regular intervals to see if any of the items have arrived on approval. When it becomes clear that a book is not coming on approval, it can be firm ordered. The disadvantages to this system are the time involved in maintaining and checking such a file and the delay that occurs when a firm order must eventually be sent for something that never arrived on approval.

Some approval plan vendors offer a better method of handling these situations. These vendors allow their customers to preview each approval batch prior to shipment by means of online access to the vendor's computer. There, the list of books selected to arrive in the next approval shipment can be viewed, as well as those excluded by the library's approval profile. These selections and exclusions can then be modified online by the library before the items are shipped. For example, if the library just received a book as a gift, it can be deleted from the forthcoming approval shipment. Conversely, if a title has been excluded by virtue of its format or publisher, and the library nevertheless wants it, the library can override the exclusion. By previewing the approval batch, book selectors can also make preliminary judgments on individual titles and eliminate items definitely not wanted, thereby reducing the number of books that need to be returned. Previewing is a powerful feature and will probably be offered by most vendors in the future.

Another area of approval plan management in which acquisitions and collection development operations must be coordinated is the handling of books not selected and returned to the vendor. In many automated systems, individual acquisitions records can be annotated to show the reason for a book being returned. A printout of these records at regular intervals can guide collection developers in reshaping the approval profile. For example, certain publishers' books or certain publication formats may be consistently returned, indicating that they should probably be eliminated from the profile. Even in a manual system, it is worth the effort to annotate approval book records with the reason for their return.

Ongoing evaluation of vendor performance is at least as important for approval plans as it is for firm orders. Both qualitative and quantitative data should be collected on the regularity and completeness of shipments, the accuracy of invoices, the physical condition of shipments, and the ability of the vendor to solve problems.

Vendor Evaluation

Acquisitions librarians and paraprofessionals make unconscious evaluations of their book vendors almost every day, with every single contact. While these subjective evaluations are useful, objective evaluations involving data collection and data analysis are essential. For most libraries, monograph acquisitions account for a significant portion of the annual budget, and acquisitions managers need to ensure that this money is spent in the most efficient manner possible. Four factors are commonly considered when evaluating a vendor: fulfillment rate, speed, discount, and service [9].

Many automated systems can provide summary calculations relevant to the first three factors, and even a manual system can provide this information without too much difficulty. The fourth factor, service, is a subjective and qualitative factor, which can be difficult to measure. However, the library staff who communicate directly with the vendor should be queried regularly to monitor service levels. Do they find that the vendor solves problems with minimal follow-up? Do they find the vendor's reports useful and complete? In addition, specific instances of vendor error (e.g., incomplete order, wrong price, wrong book, defective book) can be tracked and quantified. The American Library Association has published the *Guide to Performance Evaluation of Library Material Vendors* [10], which gives examples, procedures, and pitfalls in conducting vendor performance evaluation. Other methods by individual libraries have been well described in the literature [11-13].

Evaluation should be considered a two-way street. It is very helpful to check with vendors regularly to find out if there is anything that the library is doing that is making the vendor's job more difficult. Sometimes relatively minor changes in procedures or policies can make life much easier for the vendor and result in better service for the library.

Direct Orders

Some publications are not available from vendors and must be firm ordered directly from the publisher. In library jargon, these firm orders are called "direct" orders. For example, many publications of professional associations are not available through book vendors. Publishers of these books may not have business relationships with book vendors for a variety of reasons, including a requirement for prepayment, an unattractive or nonexistent discount structure, or simply because the publisher feels the need for a direct relationship with its library customers. Book vendors usually provide their customers with a list of publishers they can handle. If a publisher is not on the vendor's list, the library will probably need to order directly from the publisher.

There are also special cases in which it may be preferable from the library's perspective to order from a publisher instead of a vendor. Sometimes a publisher may offer a special sale on its publications, with a discount exceeding that of the vendor. Or, a book may be required in a hurry, and experience may indicate that the publisher can supply it faster than the vendor. While using a book vendor offers many conveniences, the library should not hesitate to place a direct order when this method can get the material faster or cheaper.

When placing a direct order using information from a publisher's announcement or catalog, close attention should be paid to any special ordering requirements. While the list price of a book can be obtained from other sources, such as *BIP*, the announcement or catalog provides information about other possible expenses, such as shipping and handling charges, or sales tax. Some publishers require prepayment for all orders, while other publishers only require individuals, not institutions, to prepay. Many publishers, however, eliminate shipping and handling charges if the order is prepaid. If a prepaid order is being placed based on bibliographic information only, any special requirements or extra charges should be confirmed with the publisher first, to prevent over- or underpayment.

To avoid potential problems with direct orders, libraries may find it easier to substitute or accompany their order forms with a cover letter that includes title-specific order information as well as general information on invoicing and shipping requirements. For prepaid orders it is essential that a copy of the order or other "remittance advice" accompany the check, indicating exactly what is being ordered and where the order should be sent. The library may need to work with the institution's Accounts Payable department to ensure that checks are accompanied by adequate documentation of the order.

Prepayments may also require calculation of applicable state sales taxes. In most cases, information on sales tax is included on the publisher's order form. While some states require all but government agencies to pay state sales tax, in other states libraries in educational or other nonprofit institutions may also be exempt. Most tax-exempt institutions have a certificate that can be sent along with orders to confirm the institution's tax-exempt status.

Ordering from Societies and Associations

Although a few of the larger professional societies, such as the American Medical Association and the American Psychological Association make their publications available through biomedical book vendors, most society publications must be ordered direct, and many societies require prepayment, even from institutional purchasers. Two additional wrinkles in obtaining society publications are the availability of deposit accounts and special pricing for member institutions.

Deposit Accounts

Depending on the clientele a library serves, the acquisitions department may find itself ordering almost all of the publications produced by a scientific or health professional association. For example, libraries serving nursing schools probably purchase almost everything published by the National League for Nursing (NLN). Ordering these publications individually would consume a large amount of staff time. However, the NLN, like many associations, offers a standing publication order service (sometimes called a blanket order). This service automatically sends all of the latest NLN publications to the enrolled library, at a discounted price, with free shipping and handling. To enroll in this service, a library pays the NLN a lump sum to establish a deposit account. Each month, the NLN sends the library a batch of the new publications and deducts their cost from the deposit. Periodically, the library deposits more money to maintain the deposit. This procedure can save both time and money, because no orders or invoices are required. The American Nurses Association and the American Chemical Society are examples of other associations that offer variations on this type of ordering plan.

Membership Pricing

Many associations offer special discounted pricing for their members. In some cases, these discounts are quite significant. Even though a library may not be a member of the association, several associations offer an "umbrella" discount to departments of a member institution. For example, both the American Hospital Association and the Association of American Medical Colleges offer membership discounts on their publications to the libraries of member institutions. In some cases, the book order needs only to indicate that the parent institution is a member. In other cases, the book order must include the institution's membership number to qualify for the discount.

Health Science Bookstores

Most U.S. health science schools have a biomedical book store nearby or even on campus. These stores are similar to other commercial book stores, but they specialize in carrying current health science textbooks and study aids. In general, they do not stock the foreign, expensive, or research materials often needed by health science libraries. However, many libraries find that these book stores are ideal for "rush" orders of textbooks needed for reserve or for extra copies of popular items. If these items are in stock, they can be picked up and added to the collection within hours. Although most health science book stores charge the full list price for books, it may be possible for a library to establish a regular discount if it purchases in sufficient quantity.

Acquisition of Special Materials

Microforms

In the 1960s, microforms were hailed as the future of libraries—they were cheaper to produce, more permanent, and took up less space than printed volumes. This future, needless to say, never materialized to any significant extent. A proliferation of different formats (microfiche, microfilm, microcards, positive polarity, negative polarity), sizes (16-mm, 35-mm, 24-to-1 reduction, 48-to-1 reduction), and storage media (reels, cartridges, cassettes) splintered the marketplace. Not only was it expensive for libraries to purchase all of the possible machines needed to read the various microforms, it was also onerous to maintain the machines and to train staff and clients in how to use them. Library users never became comfortable with microforms, and most of them disliked the copies produced by the wet process used by the early machines.

While it appears that advances in electronic publishing will further erode the role of microforms in libraries, there is still a niche market for them today. Monographic microforms include reprints of out-of-print books, dissertations, some government documents, and historical collections. A useful tool for verifying and ordering microforms is *Guide to Microforms in Print*, published by K. G. Saur, which serves as the *BIP* of microforms. A supplemental subject guide is also available.

Unlike microform versions of journals, most monographic microforms are available only from their producers and must be ordered directly from them. When ordering microforms, it is essential that the correct format, size, reduction ratio, and polarity are clearly indicated on the order form. The owner's manual of the library's microform reader can be checked to verify these elements.

Government Documents

A special class of publications, produced by the various units of local, state, and federal governments, are usually referred to as "government documents." Examples of these are the many publications from the U.S. Department of Health and Human Services, which are often needed by health science libraries. A few vendors specialize in supplying government documents exclusively; most general book vendors do not supply them at all.

Many U.S. federal government documents are available through the Documents Sales Service of the Government Printing Office (GPO). However, government cost reductions during the 1980s drastically reduced the number of government publications handled by the GPO. The GPO decides which government documents it will provide for sale, basing its decision on public interest and the number of copies it thinks it can sell. Because of this restriction, the majority of government documents are available only from their issuing government agency, and not from the GPO.

Before ordering from the GPO, it is wise to first confirm the price and availability of the desired item. It is also important that orders to the GPO have the GPO stock number (S/N) identified, since this is the most reliable way of identifying the unique title desired. Orders must either be prepaid (checks made payable to the Superintendent of Documents) or charged to an established deposit account. Libraries that order many items from the GPO may find establishing a deposit account the easiest method. When items are shipped, their costs are deducted from the deposit. Monthly statements from the GPO help the library to judge when to add more money to the account. In addition to its mail order service, the GPO also operates over twenty GPO bookstores. They are located in major U.S. cities, but each maintains only a small percentage of all available GPO titles, generally the most popular titles.

Order information for U.S. government documents available through the GPO is available from a variety of sources [14]:

- ***Publications Reference File.*** This bimonthly microfiche, published by the GPO, lists all of its publications currently in stock. It is arranged in three sections—by stock number, Superintendent of Documents (SuDoc) class number, and an alphabetical section of subjects, titles, and series. This file is also available online through DIALOG. Customers with GPO deposit accounts can even place orders online through DIALOG.

- ***U.S. Government Books.*** An annotated catalog of the most popular government documents, this is issued quarterly and arranged by subject category.

- ***New Books.*** A bimonthly catalog of all new titles available through the GPO, it is arranged by subject category and is not annotated.

- ***Monthly Catalog of United States Government Publications.*** Primarily a cataloging and reference tool, the *Monthly Catalog* includes documents not available through the GPO (i.e., available only from the issuing agency). It is arranged by SuDoc number, with author, title, subject, and series indexes. Complete ordering information, including the GPO Order and Information Desk phone number, is included in each issue.

Many federal agencies produce specialized publications called technical reports, which are usually not available through the GPO. These items must be ordered from the National Technical Information Service (NTIS). For example, many publications from the National Library of Medicine are available only through NTIS. NTIS maintains about two million items for sale, available in print, microform, and even electronic formats. The NTIS Bibliographic Database lists all available documents, including order information. The database is available online through several online vendors, as well as in CD-ROM format. The Database is used to produce printed publications such as *NTIS Alerts* (formerly *NTIS Abstract Newsletters)* and *Government Reports Announcements & Index*, which list newly available NTIS items.

NTIS offers a variety of ordering methods, including telephone, mail, and fax orders. Online orders can also be sent through DIALOG, OCLC, ORBIT, and STN. Payment can be made by credit card, check, money order, NTIS deposit account, or by purchase order. A standard handling fee is added to each order (not item), and an additional fee is added for each purchase order. Rush processing service is available for an extra fee. It is essential to indicate the format of the NTIS product ordered, since in many cases both paper and microfiche versions are available. Each individual NTIS title has a unique ordering number, which should be used to ensure accurate fulfillment. If this order number can't be located, it can be obtained by contacting the NTIS Identification Department.

Even though both GPO and NTIS sell thousands of documents, many government documents can only be obtained from the issuing agency. Some agencies sell their documents, while other agencies supply them free of charge. If GPO or NTIS can't supply a particular document, it is usually worth the effort to contact the issuing agency. When contacting agencies, it is always useful to ask to be added to their mailing list since many agencies automatically send out notification of new publications, or even the publications themselves, to their mailing lists. Health-related agencies that maintain mailing lists include the Agency for Health Care Policy and Research, the National Clearinghouse for Alcohol and Drug Information, and the National Center for Health Statistics.

Most state governments also produce documents that may be of interest to health science libraries, such as epidemiological statistics and public health regulations. Once identified, most of these can be obtained from the state health department, although the state health codes themselves are often printed by private publishing companies that specialize in legal publications. The Library of Congress attempts to collect all of this material, and publishes the *Monthly Checklist of State Publications* as a bibliographic guide. Every title in the checklist has full cataloging information, which should include enough information for sending order inquiries.

The World Health Organization (WHO) issues publications from both its headquarters in Geneva and from its regional offices. It also distributes publications from the International Agency for Research on Cancer (IARC), the Council for International Organizations of Medical Sciences (CIOMS), and the English language publications of the Pan American Health Organization (PAHO). Prepaid orders can be sent to WHO headquarters in Geneva, but WHO also maintains sales agents throughout the world. In the U.S., book orders should be sent to WHO Publications Center USA, 49 Sheridan Avenue, Albany, NY 12210.

Out-of-Print Books and Reprints

As scientific knowledge accumulates at an ever faster pace, health science books stay in-print for shorter periods. In addition, since federal tax laws do not encourage U.S. publishers to maintain large inventories of books, print runs have become smaller. The result is that unless a book is ordered within a few years of its publication, it is quite likely to be out-of-print when it is requested. Most libraries are still able to satisfy information needs by borrowing out-of-print (OP) books on interlibrary loan. If a library needs to purchase such a book, either for expanding the collection or to replace a missing or damaged item, there are additional options. Success rates for purchasing OP books are quite low, however, and the process can be long and expensive [15].

A common technique to acquire OP books is to publish a listing of desiderata, or "want list", in publications read by OP dealers. A library may list its desiderata at no charge in *The Library Bookseller.* For a fee, a library can list its desiderata in *Antiquarian Bookman's Weekly,* which reaches most OP dealers. Dealers who have any of the listed books then contact the library directly. A new way of publishing and searching a want list is through Interloc, a computerized service. Interloc consists of a large database of available OP books sent in by hundreds of booksellers, collectors, and dealers. For a charge, a library enters its desiderata into Interloc, which then attempts to match the individual items with those already in the database, greatly speeding up the searching process. Desiderata can even be stored in Interloc (also for a charge), in case a match shows up later. Interloc does not charge transaction fees for items bought, sold, or traded on the system. As the Interloc database grows, there should be greater chances of matches. Interloc may be contacted at P.O. Box 5, Southworth, WA 98386-0005.

A library may also wish to send its desiderata directly to OP book dealers. Many of these dealers specialize in the health sciences. Published directories [16-17] provide both geographical and subject specialty listings of OP dealers. Another option for OP books is to use search services. These are individuals or companies who take desiderata from libraries and attempt to find the items using their own contacts. In addition to the cost of the *items,* the search *service* adds on a searching fee. Advertisements for search services can be found in both *The Library Bookseller* and *Antiquarian Bookman's Weekly.*

Bypassing OP dealers and search services, the University of California at Berkeley Library reported a success rate of 24% to 36% in obtaining OP books directly from the books' authors or editors [18]. The Berkeley experience further indicates that not only does this technique work well for the sciences, but about half of the authors or editors who were able to supply items actually donated them, and the other half sold them at reasonable prices.

Obtaining reprints of OP books is yet another option. Several companies specialize in producing reprints of older books. These materials are listed in *Guide to Reprints,* an annual international bibliography of books, journals, and other materials published by Microcard Editions. UMI (formerly University Microfilms International) produces reprints of OP books in hardcover, paperback, or microfilm. Their "Books On Demand" service covers many subjects, including the medical sciences. These reprints are reproduced xerographically on acid-free paper. Subject catalogs and an author guide are available upon request from UMI, Out-of-Print Books on Demand, 300 North Zeeb Road, Ann Arbor, MI 48106.

Dissertations and Theses

Rarely, a library may need to purchase a dissertation or thesis produced at another institution. Many of these may be ordered from UMI. Over 400 institutions send copies of doctoral dissertations and masters theses to UMI, which microfilms them and produces *Dissertation Abstracts International* and *Masters Abstracts.* Both microform copies and printed copies are available for purchase. Complete ordering information and pricing is provided in every issue.

Handling of Donated Books

Accepting donated monographs and making decisions about their disposition is usually a collection development function. However, once gifts have been accepted for the collection, acquisitions records must be created before the books are passed on for cataloging. As with regular orders, gifts should be checked against both the public catalog and the on-order file to identify duplicates. If a gift will be an added copy or will replace a damaged copy, this information must be passed on to cataloging.

Most automated acquisitions systems have a gift receipt function, which creates a special gift record. These gift records are similar to regular records, but do not create an order, and will usually substitute the option of adding the donor's name and an estimated value instead of prompting for vendor and price. Libraries with manual systems may want to create a special form for gift items that will not be confused with regular orders but can be interfiled with completed orders for record keeping.

All gifts should be acknowledged in writing. The simplest method is to maintain on a personal computer a standard form letter that can be edited by inserting the donor's name, address, date, and number of books donated. For exceptional gifts of extraordinary value, a detailed description of each item should be included in the letter. Copies of gift acknowledgment letters should be kept on file for several years.

Changes in the U.S. tax law in 1984 placed added requirements on donors wishing to claim tax deductions for noncash charitable contributions. Donors of books and manuscripts to libraries must not only itemize these deductions on their tax forms, they must also supply an appraisal of any gift worth more than $5,000. This appraisal must be made by a disinterested third party, which means that the library receiving the gift is disqualified from appraising it. Experienced acquisitions librarians know that most books received as gifts consist of a box or two of vintage textbooks, with a combined value far below the $5,000 limit. Nevertheless, most libraries will not supply an estimate of the value of any gift books in their acknowledgment letters. This process not only clears the library of any legal obligations, it saves a tremendous amount of time. Because Internal Revenue Service regulations are constantly changing, acquisitions librarians need to monitor the professional literature for notices of new IRS policies affecting library donations.

Management Issues

The generally low professional regard for acquisitions-related work in libraries has led to its memorable characterization as "a vale of humility between two mountains of conceit" (i.e., collection development and cataloging) [19]. Yet, as the originator of that tag has pointed out, acquisitions work is at the core of a library's mission, contributing to both the development of the collection and to bibliographic control. To have an effective and efficient acquisitions department, however, it must be managed, not merely supervised. Effective management looks at the entire acquisitions environment and is concerned with much more than oversight of routine operations.

Combined Acquisitions/Cataloging Records

A central concept of an integrated library system (ILS) is to have a bibliographic record entered only once into the system. This means that the same record that is used to order a book is subsequently modified for use in the public catalog display. Increasingly, this record is obtained by searching a bibliographic utility such as OCLC or RLIN and then downloading the record into the ILS. Once in the computer, the acquisitions module of the ILS uses it to produce an order record, and the cataloging module uses the same record for display in the public catalog, usually with a note that the item is on-order.

This combined acquisitions/cataloging record has the potential for reducing costs and time in technical services operations. If acquisitions personnel are searching a bibliographic utility for verification, and then cataloging personnel later are searching for the same record a second time, costs for searching could be cut in half by using a combined record. Furthermore, by downloading an acquisitions record from a bibliographic utility, only the local data elements such as vendor and fund need to be keyed. A study at the University of Houston Libraries revealed an 88% reduction in keystrokes by using a downloaded OCLC record to create a single record for acquisitions and cataloging [20]. In addition, the study found an improvement in the accuracy and completeness of the bibliographic information.

Before implementing use of downloaded bibliographic records for shared acquisitions and cataloging use, consideration should be given to personnel and organizational issues. The primary questions to be answered are: Who does the searching for the bibliographic record, and who decides which record to use when multiple records are available? Since final responsibility for bibliographic description belongs to cataloging personnel, some libraries using combined records have assigned them these duties. Other libraries have successfully trained acquisitions personnel to take on these tasks. Taking advantage of the combined acquisitions/cataloging record requires new thinking from both departments [21]. In many cases, new work flow and new procedures need to be created. For example, decisions must be made on how to handle orders for items that are not found in the bibliographic utility, how and when to upgrade CIP cataloging, and at what point to add the library's holdings symbol to the bibliographic utility record.

Fund Management

Although it isn't necessary to have taken accounting courses to manage an acquisitions department, it is helpful to be familiar with basic bookkeeping principles. The acquisitions department spends a considerable portion of the library's funds, and it must take responsibility for the proper management of those funds. Because monograph acquisitions can involve thousands of individual orders, invoices, and payments in a year, managing monograph funds can require at least as much diligence as managing the library's typically larger serials funds.

While every library has different procedures for ordering, invoice approval, and payment processing, there are four basic questions that acquisitions must always be able to answer [22]:

- Allocation: How much money is there to spend?

- Encumbrance: How much money has been committed to outstanding orders?

- Expenditure: How much money has actually been disbursed?

- Free balance: How much money is left to spend?

Allocation

The amount of money available for spending each year is typically determined outside the library. Acquisitions, collection development, or the library administrative staff may submit a budget request, but the administration of the parent institution, after weighing all such requests, usually sets the amount. For some libraries, this money comes from one fund. For other libraries, the acquisitions budget may come from a combination of several funds.

Libraries may find it convenient to divide these institutional funds into smaller subaccounts, to better track purchasing patterns. For example, some libraries divide their book funds into subject or departmental subaccounts. Thus, all surgical books are purchased using the surgery subaccount. Other libraries may divide their funds by collection, such as reference, circulating, or curriculum support. Libraries that use multiple vendors sometimes set up separate funds for each vendor.

Encumbrance

An encumbrance is an anticipated expenditure based on an outstanding order. If an order is entered for a book that is estimated to cost $100, it immediately adds $100 to the library's encumbered funds. Total encumbrances must be considered along with actual expenditures in determining whether funds are available for additional purchases. Tracking encumbrances avoids the embarrassing experience of ordering $2,000 worth of books when the library only has $1,000 available.

Small libraries ordering very few books may not need to worry about encumbrances. At any one time, a small library typically has few outstanding orders, and there is little danger of serious overspending. Larger libraries almost certainly need to track encumbered funds, since at any one time they may have large amounts of money committed to outstanding orders. Encumbrances become particularly important near the end of the fiscal year, when the library needs to know exactly how much money is left to spend. Most automated acquisitions systems can automatically calculate the amount of money encumbered for outstanding orders and can unencumber money when orders are paid. It is possible to track encumbrances in a manual system, but difficult and time consuming to do so.

Expenditure

The amount paid for each item is determined from the invoice for that item, and fund expenditures represent the aggregate of such payments. Elements of expenditures that libraries may want to track separately include the list price of the items purchased, the discounts applied, and additional charges such as service fees, shipping and handling charges, and sales tax. Expenditures may be reported by account, by vendor, by type of material, or other breakdowns; monthly and year-to-date expenditures are also commonly reported. Accurate expenditure tracking also requires tracking of applied credits for returned items or other adjustments.

Free Balance

The free balance in an account is the amount of money available to spend. It is calculated by subtracting both account expenditures and account encumbrances from the account allocation. For successful operation of both acquisition and collection development functions, the accurate reporting of free balances is essential. Without close monitoring of free balances, budgets can be overspent or underspent. Overspending can have disastrous institutional consequences and at the very least damages the library's credibility. Underspending means that budgeted funds are lost, since most libraries are not able to carry leftover money into the next fiscal year. Underspending can also result in a reduced budget base for subsequent years.

Although every library requires its own breakdown of expenditures and free balances, the following categories are commonly used:

- Year-to-date expenditures, encumbrances, and free balances.

- Monthly account expenditures, encumbrances, and free balances.

- Monthly vendor expenditures, encumbrances, and free balances.

- Monthly total expenditures, encumbrances, and free balances.

- Expenditures by type of purchase (e.g., new, replacement, added copy).

Some of these categories can be combined into monthly reports that cumulate during the fiscal year. Spreadsheet programs allow even small libraries to produce presentable and informative expenditure reports. Figure 2-3 is an example of a spreadsheet produced at the end of May that shows both monthly expenditures by vendor and year-to-date expenditures. The bottom section also shows the budget allocation assigned to each vendor, the running encumbrances, and the free balance.

Forecasting Expenditures

The acquisitions department plays an important role in determining the annual acquisitions budget by providing data on current expenditure levels. Expenditure reports should be retained for several years, because they provide historical spending trends that can be used for forecasting

Monthly Expenditures by Vendor					
	Bookstore	Vendor A	Direct	Vendor B	Monthly Total
July	$0.00	$334.17	$268.83	$4,001.00	$4,604.00
August	$0.00	$252.29	$844.25	$3,653.90	$4,750.44
September	$0.00	$304.04	$66.65	$5,862.98	$6,233.67
October	$0.00	$152.51	$344.03	$5,428.20	$5,924.74
November	$34.95	$383.15	$296.02	$9,089.76	$9,803.88
December	$52.95	$69.65	$24.26	$4,860.68	$5,007.54
January	$0.00	$290.99	$145.78	$6,483.64	$6,920.41
February	$165.00	$582.18	$174.26	$10,097.62	$11,019.06
March	$0.00	$701.89	$1,569.86	$7,593.38	$9,865.13
April	$0.00	$26.96	$271.00	$2,405.60	$2,703.56
May	$0.00	$570.19	$652.59	$1,092.74	$2,315.52
June	$0.00	$0.00	$0.00	$0.00	$0.00
Allocation	$300.00	$4,000.00	$6,000.00	$70,000.00	$80,300.00
Expenditures	$252.90	$3,668.02	$4,657.53	$60,569.50	$69,147.95
Encumbrance	$0.00	$195.75	$850.00	$3,200.00	$4,245.75
Free Balance	$47.10	$136.23	$492.47	$6,230.50	$6,906.30

Figure 2-3: Sample Spreadsheet of Monthly Vendor Expenditures

future budget needs. These reports are also useful near the end of the fiscal year, when careful monitoring of expenditures is essential. By knowing how much money was spent month-by-month in previous years, good estimates can be made for the remainder of the current year.

Health science book vendors also supply annual statistics on the volume and aggregate costs of biomedical book publishing output. These reports are usually subdivided by subject and publisher, showing the number of titles and the average cost per book in each category. Although the reports are often addressed to the acquisitions department, they are very useful for collection development purposes as well.

Reports and Statistics

Requirements for reports and statistics vary from institution to institution. Many statistics are gathered and sent to organizations outside the health science library, such as the university's main library, library professional organizations, and agencies of the state or federal government. Other statistics are valuable for the internal management of the library.

Acquisitions statistics have been grouped into five functional areas [23]:

- **Quantifying load and demand.** By counting books ordered and received, invoices processed, and other activities, staffing levels can be justified. These numbers are also useful in planning for automation.

- **Identifying characteristics of order requests.** Keeping track of requests by subject or department of requester can reveal the interest of the library's clientele and the adequacy of the collection.

- **Measuring productivity.** Typical productivity categories are average time needed to complete preorder searching or to enter order information into the computer. This information can help define productivity goals or training needs.

- **Assessing performance.** Both internal and external performance can be measured. Internally, turn-around time between the order request and order placement is important. Externally, average time to fill an order and the number of claims required can assess vendor performance.

- **Assembling a financial profile.** Accurate and timely financial reports are vital for making spending decisions and doing budget planning.

Some reports are needed weekly, others monthly, and some only once a year. Most automated acquisitions systems can automatically supply a variety of reports and statistics. Some systems can provide only preprogrammed reports, while other systems allow customized reports to be produced. Libraries using manual acquisitions files should have their files organized for easy retrieval of data necessary for reports. In addition to their on-order files and items-received files, many of these libraries use data sheets that allow acquisitions personnel to tick off counted activities such as items ordered, items received, invoices processed, or claims sent out.

Other useful reports highlight vendor performance data. Many automated systems are able to calculate for each vendor the number of orders sent, number of claims sent, average delivery time, and average discount. Nonautomated libraries usually find these numbers more difficult to gather, but they are essential for evaluating vendor performance. While many types of reports can be created, the effective manager produces only the reports that are needed to make decisions, plan for the future, or fulfill external requirements for statistical reporting.

Records Management

No two libraries completely agree on the nature and extent of paper files that need to be maintained in support of acquisitions functions. Factors such as the library's size, its degree of automation, the reporting obligations of the library, and institutional requirements dictate the number and type of files needed. Generally, the more automated an acquisitions department is, the less need it has to maintain paper files. Well-designed automated systems allow inquiries based on almost any desired data field, and their report-writing modules can produce reports in minutes that would require days for manual systems, if they could be done at all.

Automated and manual files are created to track the progress of individual orders and to make needed information easily retrievable. There is no need to create and maintain a file if it is unlikely to be used at regular frequencies. An important early task of a new acquisitions manager is to analyze the function and utility of existing files. Because work flow, procedures, and personnel change over time, files that were necessary at one time may no longer be needed today. Possible files for an acquisitions department are listed below.

- **Requests to verify and order.** These have been received from the selector and are ready to enter the acquisitions process.

- **Expected on approval.** These are requests that are expected to arrive in a future approval shipment. When it can be verified that an item will not arrive on approval, it can be firm ordered.

- **On-order.** Although usually arranged by title, some libraries create a matching on-order file arranged by date to make claims easier to process.

- **Item received, awaiting invoice.** The item has been received, and is no longer on-order, but the invoice has not yet arrived.

- **Invoice received, awaiting item.** The invoice has been received, but the item has not arrived.

- **Completed orders.** These items have been received and paid for. It is convenient to start a new completed order file every fiscal year. Within the fiscal year, these records can be arranged by title, purchase order number, vendor, or account, depending on the library's needs. Copies of invoices and payment vouchers are kept here.

- **Vendor/publisher correspondence.** Arranged by supplier, this is usually correspondence dealing with problems in orders or payment [24].

Depending on the library's circumstances, many of these may be unnecessary, or additional files may be required. Automated systems can provide online or printed versions of most of them.

Unless a library is very young, there are probably old acquisitions records taking up space in drawers or boxes. For many librarians, it is an article of faith to keep any and all records for perpetuity or until space runs out. While automated systems may seem to hold the key for record management, most of them have limitations as well, depending on the system and the amount of storage space available. A good manager realizes there is a diminishing of returns in maintaining extensive files of old acquisitions records. Barring institutional requirements, completed records should be kept only as long as they are useful [25].

When deciding what records to keep, and for how long, it is helpful to keep track of why and how often staff members actually refer to any acquisitions records that are more than two years old. Based on such an examination, it should be possible to ascertain the age and types of records that need to be retained. However, individual institutions may have additional requirements for record maintenance. Many institutions perform audits at regular intervals, and they may require that certain order and payment records be kept for several years. Before changing policies for discard of older records, the advice of the purchasing or accounts payable offices should be solicited.

Choosing an Automated Acquisitions System

As mentioned earlier, selecting an automated acquisitions systems can be a difficult and complex management challenge. The computer industry is one of the fastest changing industries anywhere. Overnight, it seems, new hardware and software companies are formed, and old companies die or merge with one other. It is therefore futile here to recommend or even list available automated acquisitions systems, since some will have disappeared since this writing, and others will have arrived. Instead, this section will identify some strategies for identifying and evaluating automated acquisitions systems.

Identifying potential systems for consideration involves several approaches. A good beginning is to start with libraries that have already automated their acquisitions—what software and hardware are they using, and what do they think about their systems? It is best to poll only libraries of a similar size and scope to the inquiring library's, so that similar acquisitions needs can be reflected. If these libraries are nearby, it may be possible to arrange for a visit and a demonstration. The exhibits area of the Medical Library Association's annual meeting is invaluable for gathering information about automated acquisitions systems. Here, vendors of automated systems catering to health science libraries have brochures, live demonstrations, and sales people to answer questions. Additional automation vendors exhibit at the annual American Library Association and Special Library Association meetings.

There are several printed sources on library automation software to consult. Every December, *Library Journal* publishes a "sourcebook" issue. This annual issue is a directory of hundreds of library products and services, including both stand-alone acquisitions systems and integrated library systems (ILS). Another *Library Journal* feature is the "Automated System Marketplace," appearing every April. This article analyzes the ILS marketplace, with a review of leading systems and suppliers. Learned Information, Inc. publishes the *Directory of Library Automation, Software, Systems, and Services,* compiled by Pamela Cibbarelli. This annual publication lists microcomputer, minicomputer, and mainframe software packages. Especially useful is the listing of selected installation sites of the different products.

If the library is only interested in microcomputer-based library software, an extremely valuable resource is the list produced by the Federal Library and Information Center Committee of the Library of Congress. The list, called *CMBLS (Checklist of Microcomputer Based Library Software),* covers several library applications, not just acquisitions, and is intended to be comprehensive. Current plans are for the Committee to issue a new print edition every year, with periodic updates in electronic format available by dial-in access or through the Internet [26]. The list is indexed by category of application, company, microcomputer operating system, and local area network (LAN) compatibility. The American Library Association publication, *Library Technology Reports,* periodically publishes reviews of automated systems [27-30].

Early in the selection process, it is useful to compile a checklist of both essential and desirable features. When making this checklist, it is helpful to involve as many people in the library as possible, since most departments outside of acquisitions will eventually require some acquisitions-related information from the automated system. Useful checklists of potential acquisitions features have been published [31-32], but every library has specific requirements that will need to be added to any existing checklist. Many libraries may be required to prepare a documented list of required features to which automation vendors can respond as part of a Request For Proposal (RFP) process. Models for such RFPs have been published [33-34], and examples can be requested from other libraries.

Microcomputer Systems

Only a few years ago, the equipment necessary for an automated acquisitions system was beyond the means of all but the largest libraries. However, with the increased power of personal computers, combined with their decreasing prices, even small libraries are now capable of entering the automated age [35]. Many of the current microcomputer systems require minimal equipment, some of which may already be available in the library. Because the equipment will most likely not be used all day, everyday, for acquisitions work, it can also serve double-duty for word processing, spreadsheets, and database searching. This factor may make equipment requests easier to justify.

The relatively low cost of the equipment and software for microcomputer-based acquisitions systems is offset by some of their limitations. Most are limited in the number of records they can handle and the number of simultaneous users they can support. There is often only a limited selection of reports available. And stand-alone acquisitions applications don't integrate their data with other automated functions of a library, such as cataloging or the public catalog.

If a library can live with the limitations of a microcomputer-based system, it must then face the task of selecting a system. If the library or the library's institution has already settled on a microcomputer platform or operating system, only acquisitions systems running on that platform need to be examined. For example, a Macintosh-based library doesn't need to look at Windows or MS-DOS programs. If a local area network (LAN) is already in place, then only programs compatible over that network are eligible for consideration. If it is important that the acquisitions system interface with an existing circulation or public catalog system, that will further narrow the choices.

A library wanting a microcomputer-based acquisitions system is not limited to purchasing a ready-made turnkey system. It is possible, though not easy, for a library to create its own system using off-the-shelf software, usually a database management program. The process requires considerable expertise in both the software being used and in the acquisitions process. This is not a job for the beginner. However, there are many books and articles on adapting existing software for library use, and it is possible to build a useful acquisitions file that will handle orders, encumbrances, multiple accounts, reports, and claims. [36-40].

Minicomputer Systems

Early automation efforts in libraries required the use of large mainframe computers. Many libraries, not owning their own mainframes, had to borrow or pay for storage space and computer time from their campus computer departments. But as powerful computers grew smaller and less expensive, larger libraries have been able to purchase their own minicomputers. The power of these machines allows many functions of a library to be automated. Since so many library functions are interrelated, most libraries have focused on installing integrated library systems. A fully configured ILS typically supports acquisitions, serials control, cataloging, circulation, and public catalog functions. Some also encompass class reserve functions, interlibrary loan, and bibliographic database searching. As the name implies, integration is emphasized in these systems—the various modules usually have a common interface, and share a common bibliographic database. Selecting an ILS should involve every department in a library, since each department will need to evaluate the particular module it will use.

A current trend in ILS design is toward "downsizing" and adoption of client-server architecture, which means that the computation power needed to run the system is distributed between the central server(s) and the microcomputers located at user stations. One result is that less expensive microcomputers can replace the more expensive minicomputers now currently required for most ILS packages. Downsizing will eventually open up the world of integrated systems to smaller libraries. Another trend is the increasing use of a graphical user interface (GUI) as illustrated in Figure 2-4.

Evaluation of Acquisitions Operations

Once work flow and ordering procedures have been established and the staff thoroughly trained, many acquisitions tasks can proceed without supervisory intervention. While this may be desirable, the effective manager cannot become complacent. Periodic evaluation of all aspects of an acquisitions department should be part of the duties of the department manager. Unfortunately, evaluation is often relegated to a low priority. Heavy work loads in many libraries, combined with the urgency for rapid processing of orders, can give evaluation the appearance of a luxury. When approaching evaluation, it may be helpful to start with specific analyses, rather than attempting an overall departmental evaluation.

Evaluation of monograph acquisitions operations can be divided into a consideration of its internal and external environments. The internal environment consists not only of personnel and procedures, but also interfaces with other departments within the library. The external environment consists primarily of the relationship with the library's book suppliers.

Personnel evaluation can cover many topics, but job performance is usually of primary concern. Both the supervisor and the employee need to

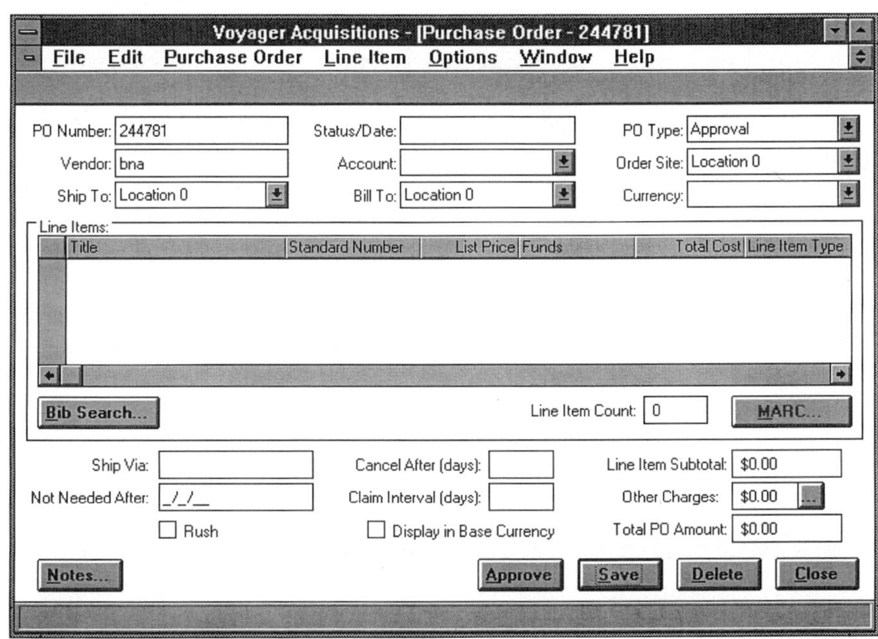

Figure 2-4: Acquisitions Screen Illustrating a Graphical User Interface (GUI) in Voyager™, an Integrated Library System (Reprinted with the permission of Endeavor Information Systems)

know how well the employee is performing. Since monograph acquisition is so heavily procedure-oriented, the ability of the employee to follow established procedures is one measure of performance. A written and consistently updated procedure manual benefits both the employee and the supervisor in establishing accepted standards of job performance.

Numeric measures are another important benchmark of job performance. Many of the statistics and reports generated during the ordering process can be used to define performance standards, such as the number of invoices processed per hour, or the number of new order entries keyed. Care must be taken, however, not to emphasize speed at the expense of accuracy. Performance standards must be realistic, combining efficiency with concern for the employee. The statistics and reports themselves should not be exempt from evaluation. Are all the statistics and reports that are produced actually used? Who uses them, and for what purposes? If the library has recently automated, manual statistics may be unnecessarily duplicating what the computer can track.

Evaluation of work flow can often be a valuable tool for increasing efficiency. Even with automated systems, there is a complex movement of people and materials in an acquisitions department. By flow charting or diagramming these movements, the librarian may discover opportunities to improve the choreography and eliminate wasteful efforts. Sometimes even a simple rearrangement of office equipment can increase efficiency. Everyone in the acquisitions department should be involved when examining work flow, because support staff often have a more immediate knowledge of work flow glitches than do their supervisors.

Acquisitions operations interface with many other functional areas in the library, and personnel from other departments should be queried regularly to determine whether the acquisitions unit is adequately responding to their needs. It is especially useful to solicit evaluation of the unit's accuracy and efficiency from the staffs of the collection development and cataloging departments.

Future Trends in Monograph Acquisitions

The forecasts of a paperless future have grown less insistent in recent years. Printed books will probably always be with us, and libraries will always need to purchase them. But there can be little doubt that their numbers will decline as electronic alternatives to the book become common. How libraries will acquire and pay for this new electronic information is the main issue affecting library acquisitions. While the debate between ownership of, versus access to, electronic information will probably go on for years, libraries require much of this new electronic information today. Acquisitions departments must be able to adapt as different methods of ordering, receiving, and paying for this information evolve [41].

New knowledge required of acquisitions librarians in the future will undoubtedly include expertise in:

- Computer systems, including hardware and software compatibility.

- Telecommunications, including wide-area networks, local-area networks, and the Internet.

- The ability to interpret licensing agreements and complex fee structures. As publishers develop different and creative methods to sell their electronic products, the library must choose the best method for its mission.

By adapting successfully to the electronic world, acquisitions, the oldest function in the library, will become the library's first link to the newest technology.

References

1. Boss R. Automating library acquisitions: issues and outlook. White Plains, NY: Knowledge Industry, 1982.

2. Magrill RM, Corbin J. Acquisitions management and collection development in libraries. 2nd ed. Chicago: American Library Association, 1989.

3. Paul SK. Notes on operations: EDI/EDIFACT. Libr Res Tech Serv 1995 Apr;39(2):180-3.

4. Alley B, Cargill J. Keeping track of what you spend: the librarian's guide to simple bookkeeping. Phoenix, AZ: Oryx Press, 1982.

5. American Library Association. Bookdealer-Library Relations Committee. Guidelines for handling library orders for in-print monograph publications. 2nd ed. Chicago: American Library Association, 1984. (Acquisitions guidelines no. 4).

6. Ibid., 7

7. Miller HS. Managing acquisitions and vendor relations: a how-to-do-it manual. New York: Neal-Schuman, 1992.

8. Dowd FB. Awarding acquisitions contracts by bid or the perils and rewards of shopping by mail. In: Katz B, ed. Vendors and library acquisitions. New York: Haworth Press, 1991:63-73.

9. Alsbury D. Vendor performance evaluation as a model for evaluating acquisitions. In: Cenzer PS, Gozzi CI, eds. Evaluating acquisitions and collection management. New York: Haworth Press, 1991:93-103.

10. American Library Association. Collection Management and Development Committee. Guide to performance evaluation of library materials vendors. Chicago: American Library Association, 1988. (Acquisitions guidelines no. 5).

11. Kent PG. How to evaluate suppliers with an automated system. Libr Acquis Pract Theory 1994 Spring;18(1):79-82.

12. Roberts P. How to evaluate suppliers in a manual system. Libr Acquis Pract Theory 1994 Spring;18(1):71-7.

13. Brownson CW. A method for evaluating vendor performance. In: Katz B, ed. Vendors and library acquisitions. New York: Haworth Press, 1991:37-51.

14. Morehead J, Fetzer M. Introduction to United States government information sources. 4th ed. Englewood, CO: Libraries Unlimited, 1992.

15. Miller, op. cit., 93-105

16. Buy books where—sell books where, 1994-1995. 9th ed. Morgantown, WV: Ruth E. Robinson Books, 1994.

17. American book trade directory, 1995-96. 41st ed. New Providence, NJ: Bowker, 1995.

18. Barker JW, Rottman RA, Ng M. Organizing out-of-print and replacement acquisitions for effectiveness, efficiency, and the future. Libr Acquis Pract Theory 1990 Summer;14(2):137-63.

19. Hewitt JA. On the nature of acquisitions. Libr Res Tech Serv 1989 Apr; 33(2):105-22.

20. Rollins G. Creating bibliographic records in the Geac acquisitions module efficiently. Libr Acquis Pract Theory Winter;1991 15(4):427-31.

21. Killens C. Blurring the lines in technical services: a report of the ALCTS Automated Acquisitions/In-process Control System Discussion Group. Tech Serv Q 1993;11(1):61-4.

22. Kruger B. Basic acquisitions accounting. In: Schmidt KA, ed. Understanding the business of library acquisitions. Chicago: American Library Association, 1990:261-85.

23. Hardy ED, ed. Statistics for managing library acquisitions. Chicago: American Library Association, 1989. (Acquisitions guidelines no. 6).

24. Ford S. The acquisition of library materials. Rev. ed. Chicago: American Library Association, 1978.

25. Eaglen A. Buying books: a how-to-do-it manual for librarians. New York: Neal-Schuman, 1989.

26. Federal Library and Information Center Committee, Library of Congress. CMBLS: Checklist of microcomputer based library software. 3rd ed. Washington, DC: Library of Congress, 1993. Available by FTP: ftp.loc.gov Directory: /pub/flicc File: cmbls30.txt or cmbls30.w51

27. Mathews JR, Parker MR. Microcomputer-based automated library systems: new series, part 1. Libr Technol Rep 1993 Mar/Apr;29(2):149-302.

28. Mathews JR, Parker MR. Microcomputer-based automated library systems: new series, part 2. Libr Technol Rep 1993 May/Jun;29(3):309-452.

29. Saffady W. Integrated library systems for minicomputers and mainframes: a vendor study, part I. Libr Technol Rep 1994 Jan/Feb;30(1):5-150.

30. Saffady W. Integrated library systems for minicomputers and mainframes: a vendor study, part II. Libr Technol Rep 1994 Mar/Apr;30(2):157-323.

31. Boss R, Harrison S, Espo H. Automating acquisitions. Libr Technol Rep 1986 Sep/Oct;22(5):479-634.

32. Duval BK, Main L. Automated library systems: a librarian's guide and teaching manual. Westport, CT: Meckler, 1993. (Supplements to Computers in libraries no. 64).

33. Boss R. Technical services functionality in integrated library systems. Libr Technol Rep 1992 Jan/Feb;28(1):5-109.

34. Boss R. The procurement of an automated library system with a model RFP. Libr Technol Rep 1994 May/June;30(3):331-439.

35. Mandelbaum JB. Small project automation for libraries and information centers. Westport, CT: Meckler, 1992. (Supplements to Computers in libraries no. 28).

36. Neill C, Callaway A, Algermissen V. Creation of a book order management system using a microcomputer and a DBMS. Libr Software Rev 1985 Mar/Apr;4(2):71-8.

37. Talley MD, McNitt VA. Automating the library with askSam: a practical handbook. Westport, CT: Meckler, 1991. (Supplements to Computers in libraries no. 43).

38. Shuster HM. Microcomputer based inhouse acquisitions program. In: Dykeman A, Katz B, eds. Automated acquisitions: issues for the present and future. New York: Haworth Press, 1989:235-62.

39. Wineburgh-Freed M, Karasick AW, Morse DH. Library-wide use of a dBase acquisitions system. Bull Med Libr Assoc. 1988 Jan;76(1):73-4.

40. Beiser K. Essential guide to dBase IV in libraries. Westport, CT: Meckler, 1991.

41. Saunders LM. Transforming acquisitions to support virtual libraries. Inf Techol Libr 1995 Mar;14(1):41-6.

3

Serials Acquisitions

Daniel H. Jones and Judith C. Wilkerson

Serials are the core of health science library collections. They represent a significant and recurring financial commitment for the library, and present complex but predictable management challenges. Current practice in managing serials acquisitions in health science libraries varies widely in terms of individual procedures, but the general outlines follow common patterns. Most libraries, for instance, establish business relationships with serials vendors to handle orders and payments to publishers. Also, computers are almost universally used, at least in larger collections, to manage serials more effectively and to provide current information about the library's collection to its users. Unique local circumstances may require unique solutions, but an examination of current practice in health science libraries reveals that standard approaches to serials acquisitions problems are widely employed.

The objective of this chapter is to provide an overview of the characteristics of serials in the health science library and to describe current practices used by libraries to acquire and control them. The availability of automated systems in support of serials acquisitions activity is now pervasive in biomedical libraries and is treated as such in this chapter. However, the basic principles underlying manual methods of ordering and receiving will also be discussed where appropriate. The terms "serials acquisitions" and "serials control" will be used here synonymously to denote the full range of procedures required to obtain and process the serials literature.

Several other chapters in this volume and in other volumes of the *Current Practice* series bear directly on issues of serials acquisitions. Matters related to selection, deselection and collection evaluation of serials are discussed in Volume 4: *Collection Development and Assessment in Health Sciences Libraries.* Postacquisition activities such as binding, handling of errata, disposition of duplicates, and union listing activities are covered in this volume in Chapter 4, Serials Management Issues. Issues relating to serials in electronic formats are examined in Chapter 5, Acquisition of Audiovisual and Digital Media.

Role of Serials in the Health Sciences and in the Health Sciences Library

In contrast to books, serials provide a rapid channel for the dissemination of information on specific topics. For this reason, they are ideally suited to the kinds of information exchange required by the volatile and highly specialized arena of biomedicine. Biomedical serials fully exploit the flexibility of the serials format, embracing a wide range of communication objectives, from the clinical case study to the review article, from the highly structured clinical trial report to the preliminary finding from the laboratory bench. By their nature, serials have an immediate impact on the work of the research communities to which they are addressed, and in this regard they are essential to the reporting and monitoring of biomedical research advances. In addition, the widespread availability of the MEDLINE database and related user-friendly search systems have made the biomedical serials literature much more accessible to researchers and students than it was even a relatively short time ago. For all of these reasons, health science libraries without exception depend on a strong and well-organized collection of biomedical serials.

The importance of serials in biomedical libraries has financial implications as well. It is not uncommon for a health science library to spend eighty percent of its collection budget on serials and for serials costs to exceed thirty percent of the library's total operating budget [1]. For this reason, the budgetary effect of continuing annual price increases, as illustrated in Figure 3-1, can be profound and must be anticipated in planning and managing the library budget. In addition to constituting a large percentage of the budget, serials subscriptions require a sustained commitment of funds over many years in order to prevent unacceptable gaps and broken runs.

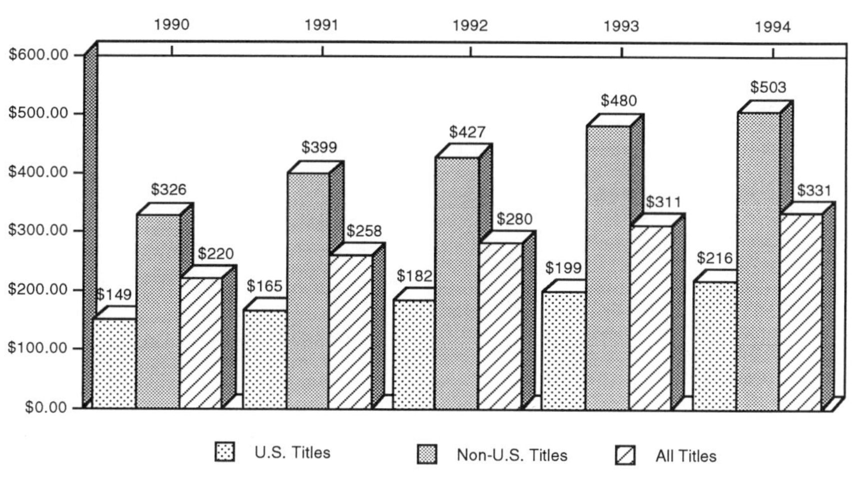

Data source: Anonymous. Price projections for 1995 subscriptions. At Your Service [EBSCO Subscription Services] 1994 Mar-Apr; 28:3.

Figure 3-1: Biomedical Journal Price Changes, 1990-1994

Categories of Serials Publications

Serials are commonly divided into two broad categories: periodicals and nonperiodicals [2]. These categories can be further subdivided but it is important to remember that these categories are somewhat arbitrary, and that many serials do not fit comfortably into any accepted taxonomy.

Periodicals

Periodicals are serials that are intended to be published on a regular schedule and are generally paid for in advance. They include scholarly journals, popular magazines, newsletters, and looseleaf publications with a regular updating service.

Journals

Journals constitute the majority of periodicals in the health sciences library. They arrive on a regular schedule (most typically weekly, monthly, bimonthly, or quarterly), usually are distributed unbound, bear a volume and issue number, and have continuous pagination throughout the volume. A volume index and cumulated table of contents are common. Journal subscriptions are usually on a calendar year basis, and a large portion of the subscriber base is made up of libraries. Journals tend to be scholarly in nature and include articles that have been peer reviewed. Examples include *Annals of Internal Medicine, Cell,* and *Image: Journal of Nursing Scholarship.*

Magazines

Magazines are comparable to journals in publication patterns but usually are intended for a wider audience. Advertisements are interspersed with articles, each issue is paged independently, indexes are uncommon, and article content is generally not subject to peer review. Magazines are usually relatively inexpensive or free. A subspecies, the controlled-circulation magazine, is published for free distribution to individual professionals in the field, but libraries may be required to pay for them. Biomedical controlled-circulation magazines are usually supported by advertising revenue or by a pharmaceutical manufacturer. Some professional societies, such as the American Diabetes Association, publish both scholarly journals and more popular magazines aimed at patients and their families. Examples of magazines commonly received in health science libraries include *New Physician, Modern Healthcare,* and *RN.*

Newsletters and Newspapers

Newsletters and newspapers are similar to journals in that they are published on a regular schedule and usually bear some form of enumeration. They are typically composed of folded sheets and frequently lack standard journal features such as a table of contents and index. They are not intended to report new research but instead may function as a current alerting service. Often they are produced by small independent publishers, professional societies, or governmental agencies. Examples include *American Medical News, HIV/AIDS Surveillance,* and *Drug and Therapeutics Bulletin.*

Looseleaf Publications

Looseleaf publications are represented in health science libraries by several popular clinical texts, such as *Scientific American Medicine* and

Duane's Ophthalmology, that are issued in looseleaf format and are updated regularly with additional or replacement pages for an annual fee. "Issues" of replacement pages frequently have a numeric designation that helps the library determine that all updates have been received. Many of these publications are also offered as CD-ROM subscriptions.

Nonperiodical Serials

There is little agreement as to what constitutes a nonperiodical serial. Librarians, publishers, and vendors sometimes use the same words with different meanings in describing them. In libraries, these titles are frequently referred to as "standing orders," while vendors and publishers may put them in a category they called "continuations." Common characteristics are that they are issued somewhat irregularly and are not paid in advance, but rather are billed at the time that they are actually supplied to the library. Libraries typically enter a "standing order" with the publisher or, more commonly, with a vendor to receive new volumes as they are published. Nonperiodical serials encountered in health science libraries include annuals and numbered series.

Annuals

Annuals are titles published on a more or less yearly basis. They can provide updating reviews of the literature in a specific discipline (e.g., *Year Book of Hematology, Annual Review of Nursing Research*), compilations of standard data (e.g., *Hospital Statistics, Physicians Desk Reference*), directory information (e.g., *Directory of Graduate Medical Education Programs, AHA Guide to the Health Care Field*), or proceedings of annual professional meetings.

Numbered Series

Numbered series include booklike publications that are issued with a collective series title and consecutive volume number, frequently but not necessarily accompanied by a unique title for each work in the series. Volumes are generally published on an irregular schedule and, after check-in as serials, are considered for separate monographic cataloging if volumes bear individual titles and authors. Although the volumes may actually be added to the book collection, order records are generally maintained in the serials acquisitions files of the library because, like other serials, a single order results in a continuing series of receipts.

Pseudoserials

Other types of publications also fit the description of nonperiodical serials for acquisitions purposes even though they are not strictly speaking serials. Encyclopedias and other multivolume works are sometimes issued one or two volumes at a time over an extended period of time. Because these publications have a defined endpoint, they are not true serials, but the ordering and receiving procedures are similar to those for other types of serials standing orders. Successive editions of standard textbooks or reference works can also sometimes be handled as standing orders through book or journal vendors. Examples include titles such as *Harrison's Principles of Internal Medicine* and *The Merck Index*.

Publishers of Biomedical Serials

Commercial Publishers

The typical serial in a health science library is a journal published for health care practitioners or biomedical scientists by a commercial publisher or professional society. Many health science serials are published by a small group of commercial scientific-technical-medical (STM) publishers that specialize in producing scholarly scientific journals. Some notable STM journal publishers based in Europe are Elsevier, Springer-Verlag, Karger, Munksgaard, Oxford, Cambridge, and Blackwell. Some primarily American STM journal publishers are John Wiley, Marcel Dekker, Lippincott, Raven, Plenum, Williams & Wilkins, Aspen, Mosby, and Saunders.

Although the commercial STM publishers are often criticized for the high prices they sometimes charge their library customers, they do provide a range of subscription-related services that are useful to libraries. For example, they understand that libraries need to examine sample issues before making a purchase decision, and usually provide them at no charge. They know that libraries place an emphasis on complete holdings, and establish standard terms for claiming missing or damaged issues of journals and for purchasing back issues.

Society Publishers

Another important group of players in biomedical journal publishing is the learned or professional societies. Society publishers are more common in North America than in Europe, where the tradition has been for professional society journals to be published by commercial publishers. Among the best known society-produced titles are *The New England Journal of Medicine* published by the Massachusetts Medical Society, *Science* published by the American Association for the Advancement of Science, and *JAMA* published by the American Medical Association. These periodicals are published by professional associations for the membership of the association and for broader distribution to the scientific community. The larger societies usually employ experienced publishing professionals to manage the production and distribution of their journals, and they are comparable to the commercial STM publishers in their fulfillment of library subscriptions.

The smaller society publishers are not necessarily comparable to either of the above groups, since they typically depend on small staffs who may not be familiar with standard publishing practices and the needs of library subscribers. For this reason, their publications can pose challenges to standard library acquisition methods. Common problems libraries experience with publications from these publishers include misnumbering of issues, frequent changes of address, delays in publication, and failure to correctly record orders and payments.

Governmental Agencies

Government agencies constitute another important group of serials publishers. Among the most familiar governmental serials in the health sciences library are *Index Medicus* and the annual *Cumulated Index Medicus* produced by the National Library of Medicine and available from the Government Printing Office (GPO), and the various *Medical Subject Headings* (MeSH) publications issued by the National Technical Information Service (NTIS). Other documents such as the *Clinical Practice Guideline* series from the Agency for Health Care Policy and Research are equally important. While most of these publications are inexpensive to purchase, they can be a challenge to identify and receive in a prompt and reliable manner. Libraries can enter some subscriptions directly with GPO and NTIS, but many publications are available only through the notably unreliable mailing lists maintained by the individual issuing agencies. Standing orders for irregular titles may necessitate the services of a specialist vendor to ensure receipt [3].

Acquisitions Challenges Posed by Serial Publications

Regardless of the type of serial or the nature of the issuing agency, all serials behave in ways that are not entirely predictable. In fact one of the defining elements of serials acquisitions is that, unlike a single book order, the library never completely knows what it will receive in return for its subscription payment or standing order. It can therefore be difficult for the library to determine if its receipts of a given title are in fact complete. Although a surprising number of serials maintain completely regular publications patterns over a course of decades, a substantial percentage of titles in any given year will change in some way that will pose a challenge to library procurement procedures and record keeping. Typical challenges include title changes, change of publisher, frequency changes, combined issues, issuance of supplements and other specially numbered (or unnumbered) issues, and delayed publication schedules.

Title Changes

The value of a consistent title from year to year in maintaining a serial's identity and reputation is obvious, and most health science publishers change the titles of their serial publications only when there is a corresponding change in their content or intended audience. Reasons for title changes are not always explained, but when they are given they usually include one of the following:

- Change in editorial board, sponsoring organization, or publisher.

- Response to new concepts or terminology in the field.

- Change in subject scope or targeted audience.

- Change in language, frequency, or peer review status.

Titles can also change for largely promotional reasons. For example, many titles formerly in Latin or German have in recent years been changed to English to promote a wider readership. Impending title changes frequently are announced in the journal itself and occasionally in other communications to subscribers and to subscription agents. STM publishers usually plan them to coincide with a new volume or new subscription year. Nevertheless, mid-volume title changes also occur and present special problems for binding and shelving operations [4].

Some title changes are unintentional, usually resulting from an action on the part of a cover designer. For example, if a cover and title page are redesigned, and an abbreviation or acronym for the title becomes sufficiently prominent, it may be necessary to catalog the journal under a new title. Because not all title changes can be anticipated, it is important to have procedures in place to identify them upon receipt and to handle them promptly.

Changes in Publication Pattern

Most journal publishers try to plan a full year of the journal well in advance. Included in their projections are the costs of marketing, paper, printing, and distribution. In consultation with the editor and the journal's production staff, they project the number of pages to be published in the next year. From these consultations they determine if the frequency of issues or number of volumes needs to change; then they set the price for the journal. Much of this planning occurs early in the year prior to publication of the volumes under consideration [5]. Sometimes, however, the flow of incoming articles is not correctly anticipated. If a journal receives more manuscripts than expected, rather than delay publication until the next year, the publisher may elect to publish an additional volume for the year. Additional volumes are usually supplied to subscribers for an additional charge. In response to complaints from libraries and serials vendors, STM publishers have in recent years reduced their dependence on this practice.

Supplements

Special issues, usually designated as supplements, are a common adjunct to many biomedical journals. Journals that do not routinely publish supplements may simply call them special issues. Supplements frequently contain special reports, abstracts of conference proceedings, the program for a society's annual meeting, or the annual membership directory of the sponsoring society. Supplements frequently are included in the annual subscription price for a journal, but in some cases they may need to be ordered separately at additional cost. Journal supplements that include articles on drug therapy and for which the publication costs have been underwritten by pharmaceutical companies can create special acquisitions problems, since their distribution in the United States may be legally restricted due to Food and Drug Administration regulations on pharmaceutical advertising [6].

Delayed Publication

Most journals attempt to publish on a regular schedule, but reality sometimes interferes with good intentions. Unanticipated competition for articles from rival journals, a sick or distracted editor, conflict on the editorial board or in the sponsoring society, or any number of other factors may result in a journal falling behind schedule. Serious and protracted delays in publication are often an early warning sign that a journal is headed for demise. To avoid paying for issues that may never be published, libraries often choose to advise their vendors to suspend paying further subscription charges until a journal resumes its normal publishing pattern.

Role of the Serials Acquisitions Staff

The library's serials acquisition staff is responsible for assuring that the overall goals for serials acquisitions are attained. These goals are

- To ensure that all orders are correctly placed and recorded.

- To ensure that all subscriptions are current and paid.

- To ensure that all issues belonging to those subscriptions are received and recorded.

- To ensure that issues and volumes are correctly labeled for shelving.

- To ensure that all of these goals are accomplished in the most cost-effective manner.

The serials acquisitions staff is responsible for noting any changes to a serial that might require revised cataloging and for initiating this process. They assist public services staff and sometimes users in interpreting check-in and other serials acquisitions records. They work closely with serials vendors and publishers to monitor performance and to assure that the goals of the serials acquisitions operation are met. Finally, they maintain ongoing communication with collection development staff to keep them informed of title or price changes, announcements of new titles, or any other developments that might necessitate review by serials selectors.

Role of the Serials Vendor

Commercial serials vendors, sometimes referred to as subscription agencies, provide services essential to most health science libraries. At the most basic level, the vendor accepts the library's subscription orders and forwards them to the appropriate publishers with payment. The vendor, in turn, sends the library a consolidated invoice, which the library pays to the vendor. Because the vendor has placed the order and paid the publisher, it also represents the library in communicating with the publisher when claims for skipped or late issues are necessary.

For this service the library usually pays the vendor the list price of the subscriptions plus a service fee, usually calculated as a percentage of the subscription costs. The library benefits by having a knowledgeable agent to communicate with publishers and by consolidating invoices and payments. Publishers also benefit by receiving consolidated order entry and payment from vendors, for which the vendor is in turn compensated with a discounted price from the publishers. The vendor's income is derived primarily from the difference between the discounted price it pays the publishers and the full price (plus service fee) it receives from the library.

For a variety of reasons, libraries may choose to employ the services of multiple serials vendors. Some vendors, for example, handle only standing order titles, but do so in a more reliable manner than the all-purpose subscription vendors. Also, vendors based in Europe are thought by some to offer more dependable service on journals published there than U.S.-based vendors. Given the recent instability in the serials vendor marketplace, some libraries prefer to use multiple vendors as a safety precaution. Nevertheless, it is generally understood that the number of serials vendors used by the library should be kept to a minimum in order to realize the full benefits of order and payment consolidation. Selection and evaluation of subscription vendors is a critical task in the serials acquisitions process and is discussed along with other management issues at the end of this chapter.

Serials Vendor Services

The following services provided by serials vendors are customarily covered by the service charge paid by the library.

- Place new orders with publishers.

- Notify publishers of renewals.

- Pay publishers for orders and renewals.

- Notify publishers of cancellations.

- Obtain refunds from publishers when due.

- Transfer subscriptions from previous vendors.

- Notify publishers of nonreceipt of issues, i.e., claims.

- Notify library of publisher response to claims.

- Intervene with publishers to resolve unsatisfied claims.

- Provide consolidated invoices and account statements.

- Provide information on changes of title, frequency, or publishing schedule affecting the library's subscriptions.

- Notify publishers of changes in library ship-to address.

- Provide standard statistical and fiscal reports on the library's account.

The following vendor services may be covered by the service charge, or they may be provided for an additional charge.

- Place orders for replacement issues and backfiles.

- Supply sample issues of journals.

- Provide a comprehensive catalog of published serials, either in printed or electronic format.

- Provide custom reports on the library's account.

- Provide online access to the vendor's serials information databases.

In addition, some vendors provide specialized services such as consolidated shipment of foreign publications, provision of machine-readable bibliographic records, software for automated serials control, union list products, and other automation services. The charge for these services may be handled separately or included in the service charge paid by the library. Like the service charge itself, the charges for these special services are negotiable, and libraries with large subscription accounts can expect to receive many of these services at reduced costs.

Standard reports provided by serials vendors include a regular journal status update specific to the library's orders. It may be incorporated into a report on pending claims or it may be issued separately. It provides up-to-date information on delayed issues, changes of frequency and title, cessations, additional volumes, supplements, and cumulative indexes. Vendors also generally provide periodic reports that summarize the library's serials expenditures by subject, by publisher, by country of origin, and by price category. These reports can be compiled to provide a multiple year comparison of the library's serials expenditures, and they usually can be supplied in both print and electronic formats.

Most vendors maintain an online information system that is available to their customers. Through these systems the library can communicate about orders and claims and can obtain bibliographic information from the vendor. Network links allow the vendor to transmit reports and invoice data directly to the library's computer system and can provide a gateway to other network resources.

A key person in the success of the vendor-library relationship is the account executive, sometimes called the customer representative. Most vendors designate an account executive on their staff to coordinate services for the library's account. This provides the library staff with a specific person with whom they can discuss the library's needs and concerns. Account executives generally work in teams so that a second individual is familiar with each account and can handle it when the primary account representative is unavailable. The account executive should be available to the library by telephone, e-mail, and fax, and should respond in a timely manner to the library's queries. It is the account executive's responsibility to see that the library's instructions are carried out promptly and accurately by the vendor and to advise the library on the progress of its orders, renewals, claims, cancellations, and other concerns. The account executive should work closely with the library staff to assist them in fully exploiting the service offerings of the vendor.

The Library Serials Control System

The serials control system is the library's memory of what has been ordered, paid, received, and expected. Long before computers were ubiquitous, libraries developed sophisticated manual record systems to keep track of serials orders and receipts. As computers have become more commonplace and affordable, numerous automated serials control systems have been developed to support this function.

Automated Systems

Automated serials control systems provide substantial advantages and efficiencies over manual systems in managing the ordering, receiving and payment of library materials. They typically accommodate multiple simultaneous users, both inside the library and from remote sites, and provide rapid access to records by title, keyword, and other identifying elements such as the ISSN. They can display current receipt information and summary holdings, both for the public and for staff, and provide automatic prediction of the next expected issue. Based on these prediction algorithms, automated systems permit routine claiming of skipped or delayed issues. They can accept electronic invoice information and create printed listings and online reports in a variety of formats. In addition, they can support related functions such as binding, routing, and union listing. When they are part of an integrated library system, the circulation status of individual items can be displayed in the online public access catalog.

Automated serials control systems vary from flat database files to serials modules of integrated library systems, with systems available for mainframe computers, minicomputers, and microcomputers. Some systems operate only on one type of computer and within only one operating system, while others can operate on a range of platforms. A lack of consistency in design as well as a lack of standardization in many aspects of serials control has resulted in a wide variety of functionality for automated serials control systems.

Developers and marketers of serials control systems include libraries, serials vendors, and commercial software producers. Identifying the major players is relatively easy, since most vendors of computer-based library systems with serials control functions exhibit at national and regional library association meetings. In addition, *Library Journal* regularly publishes a review of the automated systems marketplace that profiles the systems and includes a directory of names and addresses for each [7]. Another annual survey of automated systems is published in ALA's *Library Systems Newsletter* [8]. Although these reviews do not address specific functional features, they can serve as a good starting point in identifying systems that are available. *Library Technology Reports* has published studies of automated systems that address specific serials control requirements and the ability of the various available systems to fulfill them [9-10]. Other recent issues of *Library Technology Reports* have addressed serials control functions as part of a comprehensive evaluation of integrated library systems for microcomputers, minicomputers, and mainframes [11-14].

Some serials subscription vendors have applied their experience with serials and libraries to develop stand-alone microcomputer-based serials control systems, normally marketed only to their own subscription clients. The most familiar of these are REMO, developed by Readmore, Inc., and Microlinx, developed by The Faxon Company. Installation of these systems can be surprisingly simple, since the vendor can load the library's bibliographic and payment records into the system. In addition to assisting with setup of the system, the vendor can provide manuals, consultation, and training for staff. Since these systems are usually not based on MARC bibliographic records, they can present challenges if the library decides later to migrate to a system that is MARC-based. Also, because they were developed originally with staff use in mind, they may not be suitable for access by the public. Figure 3-2 illustrates a check-in screen from the REMO system.

REMO CHECK-IN SCREEN

```
                                                              Ship-to:  A15404
045469400                                                     Copy #:  001 of 1
AMERICAN J OF GASTROENTEROLOGY                                Abstr:    AMEJGA
                                                              ISSN: 0020-9270

 Freq: M            Maxvol:           Maxis: 12        Source: Readmore    0 RTG recip(s)
 Circu: REF ONLY    Status: ACTIVE    Claim Mode: SEMI-AUTO                2 TOC recip(s)
```

LN	DATE	CYR	VOL	ISS	STAT	REAS	CLM #/*	REMARKS
3	03/16/94	94	89	3	R			MARCH 1994
4	04/20/94	94	89	4	R			APRIL 1994
5	05/18/94	94	89	5	R			MAY 1994
6	06/15/94	94	89	6	R			JUNE 1994
7	07/11/94	94	89	7	R			JULY 1994
8	08/11/94	94	89	8	EXP			
9	09/11/94	94	89	9	EXP			
10	10/11/94	94	89	10	EXP			

```
Text comment:
Cur. Iss. Loc:
NOT BOUND/Bind at:
```

```
F1=Help      F2=options        PgUp/Dn=scroll up/dn      Ctrl-PgUp/Dn=go to first/last pg
H=header     F9 or Shift-F9 or Ctrl-F9 or F10=save       Ctrl-Q or Ctr-B or Esc=no save
                              Type an option then press <Enter>:
```

Figure 3-2: Screen Display from Readmore's REMO Serials Control System (Courtesy of Readmore, Inc., New York, NY)

Specific functional criteria to consider in selecting and evaluating automated systems are discussed in detail at the end of the chapter.

Manual Systems

The most common manual record system for serials control uses removable cards filed alphabetically by title in sliding file trays. The cards holders can be flipped up on hinges, allowing orders and receipts to be recorded without removing the cards from the trays. The cards themselves are formatted in a calendar-like fashion so that receipts can be recorded in the appropriate chronological block and so that any skipped issues are obvious upon visual inspection of the cards. Libraries typically add markings to the check-in records to indicate issues that have been bound.

There should also be room on the cards for processing notes, routing instructions, a summary statement of the library's holdings, and payment information. Preformatted cards for monthly, weekly, and annual serials are available from most library supply companies.

Serials Acquisitions Procedures

Procedures for order and receipt of serials represent extensions of the same basic techniques that are employed in book acquisitions, especially in such areas as communication with selectors, preorder verification, and fund accounting, all of which are introduced in Chapter 2: Monograph Acquisitions. However, many libraries still find it useful to keep monograph and serials acquisitions responsibilities almost completely divided, with separately assigned staffing for each. In the discussion of the major serials acquisitions procedures that follows, emphasis is placed on those aspects that arise from the unique characteristics of the serials literature and of its avenues of distribution.

New Orders

Communication of new serials orders to vendors or publishers requires both account-level standard instructions that apply to all titles (such as invoicing requirements and delivery address) and title-specific instructions, such as the starting year and number of copies for each title ordered [15]. One of the advantages of using a subscription vendor is that standard instructions do not need to accompany every order. Elements of the standard instructions to vendors include the following:

- Ship-to address.

- Invoicing requirements including
    - Bill-to address.
    - Required number of copies of invoices and credit memos.
    - Batch vs. individual invoices.
    - Inclusion of library assigned codes such as order number and department.
    - Preferred handling of credit adjustments.

- Policy on supplements, i.e., order only as specified, order supplements automatically, advise of supplements if available.

- Renewal policy, i.e., renew until canceled or await authorization from library before renewing.

- Acceptability of multiple-year orders.

- Order confirmation requirements.

Most vendors have their own standard policies that are applied unless the library requires a variant practice. These policies are normally included in the front matter of the vendor's annual catalog of serial titles or customer service handbook. That information also generally includes the vendor's preferred format for orders, claims, and other standard communications.

Title-specific information that should be included in all orders includes title, number of copies, and start date. Additional useful information items are the beginning volume number if known, the ISSN, and the title number from the vendor's catalog.

In most libraries, a requisition or purchase order is required to initiate an order, and this order is forwarded to the vendor. If the library has multiple accounts with the vendor, the account number must also be included. Most vendors accept telephone orders, but it is advisable to follow these with confirming written orders clearly indicating that the telephone order has been placed. Larger subscription vendors can accommodate on-line entry of orders. Figure 3-3 illustrates an online order using EBSCONET Plus.

Once a new order has been placed, processes must be initiated in preparation for receipt of the issues. These generally include preparation of a preliminary check-in record, so that the journal is not confused with unsolicited publications when delivery begins, and preparation of a payment record, so that the order and later payments can be properly recorded.

Establishing the Check-in Record

Important elements of the check-in record include the following:

- Title.

- Publisher.

- ISSN.

- Frequency (e.g., monthly, weekly, quarterly), pattern of publication (e.g. number of issues per volume, number of volumes per year), and anticipated supplements.

- Vendor (and account number if there are multiple accounts).

- Vendor title number.

- Notes for labeling and marking (e.g., call number, location, security stripping).

- Other processing and special handling instructions (e.g., how often the title is bound, notes on special issues to expect, retention policy, and volumes or issues that receive monographic cataloging).

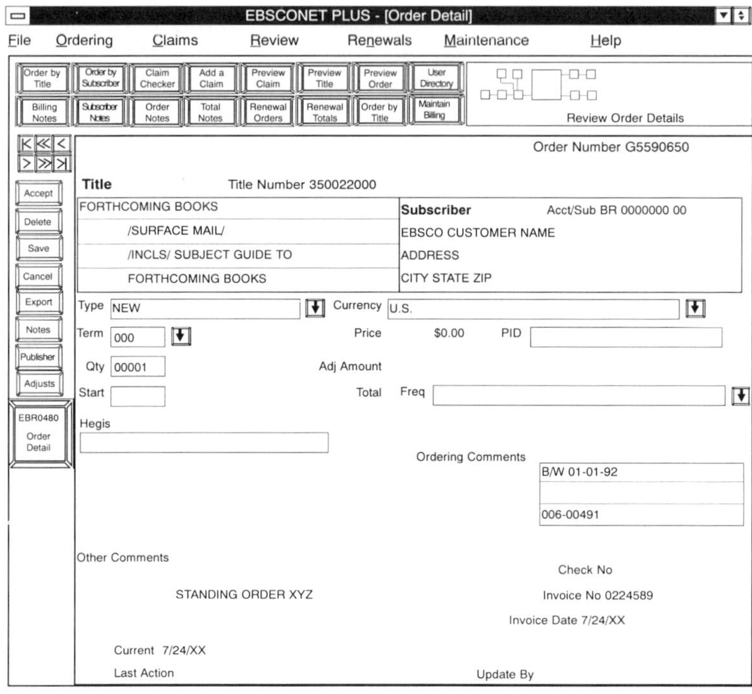

Figure 3-3: Online Order Screen Display from EBSCONET Plus (Courtesy of EBSCO Subscription Services, Birmingham, AL)

- Routing instructions.

- Order reference number, if the check-in record is not otherwise linked to the payment record.

A summary statement of the library's bound and unbound holdings of the title is usually a part of the check-in record as well. Some automated serials control systems automatically create and update this statement based on receipts and the frequency and pattern information. In manual systems and in some automated systems it must be updated whenever a volume is completed.

It may not be possible to establish all of the elements listed above until the first issue is available for examination, but as much information as possible should be included in the preliminary check-in record created at the time of order entry.

The exact title is normally established in the preorder searching process and is based on a definitive source, such as the Library of Congress or National Serials Data Program record in OCLC or other bibliographic utility, or on the SERLINE record from NLM. If the apparent cover title is different from the cataloged title, both titles should be made searchable in the check-in record. Recording of the frequency and pattern information may need to await arrival of the first issue. These publication patterns are generally described in the front matter of each issue along with other subscription-related information, such as the cost and the publisher's policy on honoring claims for missing issues.

The first issue of a new order received should be examined carefully to confirm that it is the title expected before it is passed on for cataloging. At the same time, pattern and frequency information, processing and routing instructions, and a preliminary holdings statement may need to be entered or revised in the check-in record. Union list entries and binding records may also need to be established and the library's count of current serials titles updated. In a small library all of these processes may be performed by the same person, while in a large library these tasks may be divided among several individuals. A checklist of major steps for processing the first issue of a new serial may be helpful to ensure that nothing is overlooked and that all steps are performed in the proper sequence. Figure 3-4 illustrates such a checklist. Similar procedures are involved when a journal is cancelled, ceases publication, or changes title.

Establishing the Payment Record

At least as important as the check-in record is the payment record for each title. It identifies funds encumbered for new titles not yet invoiced and provides a retrospective listing of all payments and credits for each continuing title. Such records are essential in determining that the library has not paid twice for the same volume or subscription term and in monitoring price increases. The library may use a manual system for this purpose, but an automated system offers many advantages, including the ability to summarize and analyze costs and price trends in a variety of ways. In either approach, the payment record should be linked to the check-in record so that the claiming function can be carried out with convenient access to relevant payment information.

A basic payment record includes the following:

- Journal title.

- Number of copies on order.

<u>Checklist for establishing new serials acquisitions records</u>

Title:____[ ]New subscription

____[ ]New gift serial for
                                                                          ______(yr)

Expected frequency:_________
Begin date:______________________________First issue expected:________
[ ] Title change
Previous title (Continuation of):____

	Date	Initials
Purchase order to vendor (purchasing)	______	______
or change to existing order		
For title change link to previous title		
If part of year, beginning and ending		
Bibliographic record in ILS	______	______
Source:		
Level: [ ] Basic title minimal information		
e.g., frequency, ISSN		
[ ] Full MARC	______	______
If title change: linking titles		
[ ] requires professional analysis &		
upgrade to higher level y / n		
Enter order/receipt record in ILS	______	______
Add encumbrance to fund records y / n	______	______
Add to renewal list (if separate)	______	______
or code for renewal extract tapes		
Routing / location notes	______	______
Table of contents y / n		
Retention / replacement notes	______	______
replace with fiche y / n		
New binding patterns y / n	______	______
Fiche ordered, set up y / n		
Inspect first issue received	______	______
Upgrade bibliographic record	______	______
Add MARC holdings record	______	______
Add to union list (s)		
local, regional, national	______	______
Add title to CD-ROM Reference databases	______	______
Create shelflist locations, labels	______	______
Notify selector of receipt	______	______

Figure 3-4: Sample Checklist for Establishing New Serials Acquisitions Records

- Vendor name or name and address of the publisher if ordered direct.

- Vendor account number, if multiple accounts are established for the same vendor.

- Vendor title number.

- Library fund charged.

- Ledger of payments and credits.

Every payment or credit for the title will be recorded, including the invoice number and date, the amount, and the volume(s) and year(s) covered by the payment. In automated systems the payment record for the title may be created automatically the first time that invoice data is electronically loaded. If payment records are maintained manually, it may be useful to employ color-coded sleeves or tabs to differentiate between titles purchased from different vendors or charged to different funds. Also, for those direct-order titles for which the publisher does not reliably send a renewal invoice, a calendar-based "tickler" file may be needed to remind serials staff that a periodic reorder is required.

Check-in

Check-in is the heart of serials control. Serials issues arrive at the library on a steady basis, and well-understood procedures must be in place to keep them flowing into the collection. Procedures must emphasize accurate record-keeping and efficient processing of serials as they are received by the library. There are some common problems and exceptions that can be anticipated, and procedures for handling these should be established and clearly understood by serials acquisition staff.

Efficient check-in begins in the mail room where incoming mail is sorted and prepared for distribution in the library. All mailing labels should be examined carefully so that misdirected mail is not inadvertently accepted. Some libraries keep the envelope or mailing label with each issue until it has been checked in, to assist in resolving delivery problems in case the issue turns out to be unwanted or a duplicate.

Given the time-sensitive nature of biomedical information, backlogs in mail processing and serials check-in are unacceptable. Twenty-four hours is a reasonable goal from mail receipt to availability on the shelves. Once receipt is recorded in an automated system, it is important to minimize delay in getting the issue to the shelf, since the receipt information, in many cases, is immediately available to library users.

Recording Receipt

In most automated systems, the correct check-in record can be selected by entering the ISSN or words from the title. Some automated systems can use the bar code printed on the journal to call up the corresponding check-in record. Standards for these bar codes have been established by the Serials Industry Systems Advisory Committee (SISAC). If a manual system is used, sorting receipts alphabetically before check-in can save time in moving between records. When a check-in record cannot be found for a received item, the item should be reviewed by a supervisor before it is treated as unwanted or misdirected mail.

After the correct check-in record is located, it is reviewed for notes and comments related to the issue in hand, and the issue receipt is recorded. Most automated systems display for the staff member's review the predicted volume and issue number as well as the chronological designation for the issue, based on the frequency and pattern information provided in the record. If the received item matches what has been predicted, a single keystroke can confirm that it has been received. Figure 3-5 is a screen display of a predictive check-in record in the Georgetown University Library Information System (LIS).

In a manual system the issue number and receipt date are written on the check-in record in the grid square corresponding to the volume and month of the title.

Physical Processing of Receipts

Routine physical processing of each item follows check-in. Special processing instructions may be noted in the check-in record as exceptions to routine procedures. Physical processing usually includes the following:

- Stamping receipt date.

- Stamping library name.

- Placing a mark on the cover identifying the title for purposes of alphabetic filing.

- Attaching special labels identifying locations, call numbers, or circulation status.

- Inserting a security strip.

- Attaching a bar code.

- Inserting date due slips.

```
JOURNAL:

Enter ISSN number or the initial letters of as many
words in the journal title as you wish in any order.

JOURNAL: NEW ENGLAND J MED

The New England journal of medicine.

Copy: [ 1 ] =>

                                 Checkin  Screen
The New England journal of medicine.              Copy: 1

      Is/Vl:  26     Cir loc: CURRENT JOURNALS  Bar flg: Yes
      Vl/Yr:  2      Cir sts: AVAILABLE         Bind cd:
      Freq:  W       Cir cls: THREE DAYS        Src:  Majors/Periodicals

Hold:  1928-1993  :  199-328/329N1-24/


Expected:
      Cur  yr: 1993     Cur vol: 329      Cur is: 25
      Cur  run:         Cur mon: DEC      Cur dy: 16

Enter: Y or C to confirm ; V_ N_ P_ S_ ; <ESC> ; '?' for help
```

Figure 3-5: Screen Display of a Predictive Check-in Record in the Georgetown University Library Information System (Courtesy of Dahlgren Memorial Library, Georgetown University Medical Center, Washington, DC)

Problems and Exceptions

Experienced serials staff develop a familiarity with the collection over time. As a result, they can usually recognize problem titles upon receipt. However, staff should be cautioned not to rely on memory and familiarity with the collection in processing serials receipts. The use of automated systems may make this caution even more important, since it is easy for staff to accept system-predicted issue data even though it does not match exactly what is on the piece. Similarly, staff must be alert for minor variances between the title on the piece and the check-in title, since such variances may need to be treated as title changes by cataloging staff.

Predicted receipt information generated by an automated system may be inaccurate, either because the prediction algorithm is wrong or because the publishing pattern of the title has changed. When this happens it is important to correct the underlying pattern and frequency data so that later issues will be correctly predicted. It may be useful to require higher level staff to review changes of this type.

If the issue in hand is not the next expected issue, a claim to the vendor or publisher may be necessary. An automated system should be able to recognize if one or more issues have been skipped and to identify them automatically as possible claims. In a manual system a flag may be placed in the record for follow-up review and claiming at a later time.

Another common situation encountered at check-in is the receipt of unsolicited serials. To cope with these receipts, libraries commonly maintain a disposition file to record how they should be handled when received. Disposition instructions can be kept in a separate card file, a computer database, or integrated into the check-in file. The following are examples of notes commonly used in disposition files.

- Add to samples.

- Add to exchange.

- Discard.

- Route and discard.

- Route and shelve in __________.

For unwanted publications that arrive persistently, a request to be removed from the mailing list should be sent to the publisher.

Claiming

A claim is a notification to the publisher that an item included in an order was not received or was received in unsatisfactory condition. Serials claiming relies on accurate receipt and payment records, because it is the pattern of receipt or nonreceipt that indicates that a claim is justified. Although claiming is a time-consuming activity, it is an absolute necessity if the library is attempting to maintain a reliably complete collection. Missing journal issues can have an immediate deleterious effect on patient care and research and can increase the need for interlibrary loan and public services assistance.

Elements of the Claim Notice

Claims are generally sent by the library to the vendor, which then forwards them to the publisher. Essential elements of the claim include

- Library name and account number.
- Title being claimed.
- Specific enumeration, chronology, or edition of item being claimed.
- Reason for the claim.
- Date of the claim.
- Claim sequence (e.g., first, second, third claim).

Additional elements that may be needed include

- Publisher.
- Library order reference numbers, such as purchase order number.
- Alternative identifiers for the journal, e.g. ISSN or vendor number.
- Explanatory notes.

The most common reasons for a claim are

- Skipped issue.
- Overdue issue.
- Issue damaged in transit.
- Issue misprinted, including missing pages.
- Incorrect number of copies.

Vendors usually provide preprinted multipart claim forms that include a checklist of the most common reasons for a claim. The library enters the unique information for the claim, marks the reason, and forwards a copy to the vendor. The form usually includes space to enter special circumstances not covered by the checklist of reasons. Automated serials control systems automatically produce the necessary claim letters.

Most vendors also provide online options for entering a claim. Standards that will allow automated library systems to communicate with vendors' and publishers' online systems are being developed by the Serials Industry

Systems Advisory Committee (SISAC) using the American National Standards Industry (ANSI) X12 standard for electronic exchange of business information. Among the standards in development are the order status inquiry (claims) and the order status report (claims response to agents and libraries). Automated claiming will be greatly facilitated when these standards are widely adopted by library systems and serials vendors [16].

Claiming Procedures

At least half of the battle in the claiming process is to identify the issues that need to be claimed. This process must be carried out within the time frame set by the publisher for allowable claims and before the publisher's supplies of the issue are exhausted.

In a manual system the check-in card can be flagged at check-in with a colored tab to indicate that an issue has been skipped. Flagged cards are reviewed regularly and claims to the vendor are prepared. Identifying overdue issues is more difficult since every check-in card in the file must be reviewed to determine which titles are overdue. This A to Z review must be done on a regular schedule to identify subscription and delivery problems while the missed issues are still available.

Automated serials control systems are designed to identify skipped issues upon check-in of a subsequent issue. If the item being checked-in is not the predicted next issue, the system prompts the operator to record the issue or issues that have been skipped and identifies them as potential claims. Overdue issues are identified based on the frequency of the publication, the number of days since the last issue was received, and the title-specific grace period assigned by the library. For example, a weekly may be considered overdue if no issue is received fourteen days after the most recent issue was checked in. Titles that are overdue based on this interval are flagged as potential claims by the system.

A typical schedule for claiming overdue issues based on publication frequency is indicated in Table 3-1 [17-18]. Most automated systems allow a wider range of frequencies than those listed, and generally use default grace periods for each frequency, which the library can adjust for individual titles.

Automated systems can compile all potential claims in a matter of hours or minutes, depending on the size of the check-in file. After the check-in file has been completely processed, the system usually produces a claims list that is reviewed to determine if a valid claim exists. Figure 3-6 illustrates a system-generated claims review list and detail screen as produced by Faxon's Microlinx system.

Each item on the claims list should be checked carefully against the receipt and payment files (and preferably the shelves) to verify that it is a

Table 3-1: Schedule for Claiming Overdue Receipts

Frequency	Days elapsed since last receipt
Daily	10 days
Weekly	14 days
Monthly	60 days
Quarterly	150 days
All others	30 days after expected arrival

valid claim. The availability of other libraries' serials receipt records through the Internet has provided another useful way to confirm that a missing issue has in fact been distributed to other subscribers. Once the claims review is complete, unnecessary or premature claims are deleted from the claim file, and valid claims are forwarded to the vendor or publisher.

Reducing Unnecessary Claims

Premature and unnecessary claims may be caused by the library or by the publisher. A frequent cause of unnecessary claims in libraries using automated serials systems is that the system-supplied expected receipt date has gotten off track or the grace period supplied by the system is too short. Other common reasons for libraries entering unnecessary claims include the following:

- Delayed publication not communicated to library.

- Combined issue not noticed at check-in.

- Issue checked in as supplement or on wrong title record.

- Frequency change.

- Issue received but not checked in due to human error.

- Title changes.

Common publisher errors causing unnecessary claims include the following:

- Misnumbering of issues.

```
 SUMMARY CLAIMS REVIEW                    UPDATE

                                  CLAIM                                    LAPSED
 ACT TITLE# COPY#        TITLE    ACTION          ISSUE                     ISSUES
 Y   218    1    American journal of  ↓  C1  v.74,no.3 Aug 15, 1994         Gap
 Y   232    1    Annals of internal m↓  C1  v.121,no.3 Aug 01, 1994        1
 Y   285    1    Biotechnology and bi↓  C1  v.44,no.4 Aug 05, 1994         1
 Y   290    1    Hypertension.          C1  v.24,no.2 Aug 1994             Gap
 Y   173    1    JAMA.                  C1  v.272,no.10 Sep 07, 1994       Gap
 Y   173    1    JAMA.                  C1  v.272,no.11 Sep 14, 1994       Gap
 Y   557    1    Nature.                C1  v.370,no.6493 Sep 08, 1994     Gap
 Y   65     1    Neonatal network.      C1  v.13,no.5 Aug 1994             Gap
 Y   65     2    Neonatal network.      C1  v.13,no.6 Sep 1994             Gap
 Y   45     1    Nursing standard.      C1  v.8,no.45 Aug 03, 1994         2
 Y   72     1    Proceedings of the N↓  C1  v.91,no.16 Aug 02, 1994        Gap
 Y   72     1    Proceedings of the N↓  C1  v.91,no.17 Aug 16, 1994        Gap
 Y   216    1    Science.               C1  v.265,no.5178 Sep 09, 1994     2
```

```
 CLAIMS REVIEW                TITLE#: 285          COPY     1    OF    1

 Biotechnology and bioengineering.                FREQ: semi-monthly


                                                  PATTERN: v.,no
 PUBLISHER: John Wiley                            LAPSE  : 15

 ISSN : 0006-3592          CALL#: QH324 \.B5

 SERIAL TYPE: periodical   LOCATION:              EFFECTIVE DATE:  25 Mar 91
 MEDIUM: print             ROUTE: no              PUB STATUS: curr 25 Mar 91
                           BIND : no              LIB STATUS: actv 25 Mar 91
 CURR SHELF:
 PERM SHELF:               HOLDINGS:

 SOURCE: FAXON             NOTES:

 ACT        ISSUES           DATE RCVD   LAST ACTION/DATE    COMMENTS
      v.44,no.3  Jul 1994    20 Jul 94
 C1   v.44,no.4  Aug 05, 1994
```

Figure 3-6: System-generated Claims Review Screens as Produced by Faxon's Microlinx Serials Control System (Courtesy of The Faxon Company, Westwood, MA)

- Publishing out of sequence without notifying subscribers.
- Changing frequency of publication without notifying subscribers.

There are several ways to avoid unnecessary and premature claims. Experience with claiming individual titles can be used to determine if the standard grace periods are satisfactory. Personnel doing check-in and claiming should adjust grace periods when claimed issues are repeatedly received shortly after a claim has been entered. Similarly, notes entered in the check-in record about delayed publication can aid staff in avoiding premature claims.

Titles that publish issues out of sequence can be particularly troublesome if staff are not familiar with them. Titles that are known to publish out of sequence should have a note in the check-in record to this effect, and staff should adjust the expected receipt information for these titles in order to avoid claims for the issues not received.

Some titles may not benefit from claiming at all. For example, titles with a limited retention period may be withdrawn before a claim can be resolved. A do-not-claim note in the check-in record for these and similar titles of ephemeral interest allows staff to eliminate these claims from their workload.

Follow-up Claims

Following up on unresolved claims is just as important as identifying claims in the first place. Vendors usually send to the library a monthly claim activity report, such as the one illustrated in Figure 3-6, showing the status of all claims in process for the library. These should be carefully reviewed against the library's records to determine if unfilled claims have been inadvertently dropped from the vendor's files. The reports should be checked and returned promptly to the vendor indicating which claims have been filled and which ones remain unresolved. Items still not received should be reclaimed with the vendor and recorded as such in the library's files. Responses from the vendor or publisher regarding unfilled claims should be recorded in order to document the complete claiming sequence. It is especially important to be able to document that the library's first claim notice was sent within the time period acceptable to the publisher.

Renewals

Most publishers send renewal invoices to subscribers about three or four months before the end of a subscription term. These invoices need to be paid at least six to eight weeks before the end of the subscription term to guarantee continuous delivery. Libraries commonly receive renewal notices from publishers even though the titles are ordered and paid for through a subscription vendor. Such notices can usually be ignored unless they continue to arrive past the date by which the publisher should have received payment from the vendor, typically in mid-November. In these cases, the notices should be forwarded to the vendor, with a request that their renewal be confirmed with the publisher. Needless to say, special care must be taken not to overlook renewal notices for titles that are ordered directly from the publisher.

Consolidated processing and payment of subscription invoices is one of the most important services that libraries require from subscription vendors. Especially in academic health sciences libraries, which typically maintain at least 2,000 active subscriptions, the prospect of entering and paying for renewals individually is almost unthinkable. Vendors, on the other hand, can exploit the capabilities of their automated systems to collect payments from libraries and distribute them to publishers in the most cost-effective manner possible.

Vendors generally offer two plans for renewing subscriptions, one automatic and one requiring annual reauthorization by the library. Most libraries elect to receive an annual renewal list from the vendor showing all titles on order for the library and to authorize renewals based on a review of the list. The other option is for the vendor to renew all titles automatically until instructed by the library to cancel. In either case, it is important that the library is aware of the vendor's cycle for sending renewals to publishers so that the library has adequate time to make renewal decisions. This is especially important if renewal or cancellation decisions must be coordinated with subject specialists, library committees, or other groups, either for administrative or political reasons.

The annual renewal listing is commonly issued between July and August as an invoice including all titles currently handled on behalf of the library. The library reviews the list, makes necessary changes, and returns it to the vendor with payment, usually by mid-October. Later renewal dates should be discussed with the vendor to avoid interruption of subscriptions. The renewal list includes the title, number of copies, and a price, and is accompanied by special notes about changes of title or publication schedule. Prices listed on the vendor renewal invoices frequently reflect the prices for the current year instead of the coming year, since many publishers do not finalize prices until relatively late in the year. For these titles, the vendor must follow-up later with a supplemental invoice, covering the inevitable price increases. Libraries have had some success in convincing publishers to establish and communicate their revised prices earlier in the year and in getting vendors to indicate more clearly on their invoices which prices are definitive and which are subject to supplemental billings.

Standing order titles and titles that are significantly behind in their publication schedule are generally included on the renewal list but are listed without prices. They usually have a note indicating they will be "billed later" or "billed as published."

Each title on the vendor's renewal list should be compared with the library's payment record and check-in record to make sure that the indicated renewal period is correct and that the title has not been designated for cancellation. Notes from the vendor about upcoming changes in the title or frequency should also be reviewed, since they allow the library to update check-in records in anticipation of the changes. In large libraries, renewal decisions may be made by the collection development librarian or subject specialists, while in most hospital libraries the librarian reviewing the list also makes the renewal decisions, often in consultation with the library committee. Once a renewal decision is finalized, it can be recorded in the payment record.

Renewal decisions involve one of three options: renew, cancel, or hold. The most common decision is to renew the subscription. A variant of this choice is to change the number of copies. Choosing the hold option places the responsibility on the library for renewing at a later date. It is used primarily when a title is substantially behind schedule and the library does not want to be invoiced for it until it has received what it has already paid for. It can also be used when the library needs more time to complete consideration of selected renewal decisions. When this option is exercised it is important to have a procedure for following up with final renewal decisions at a later date. In any case, clear notations on the renewal list sent to the vendor are important to avoid any doubt about the library's intentions. In addition, complex changes should be fully explained in a cover letter that accompanies the list.

Although the library generally must notify the vendor of its renewal decisions by early October, the vendor may not immediately place the order with the publisher. Vendors usually negotiate a date for order entry and payment with each of the large publishers. For calendar year publications, the date is usually in November or December. Until then, the vendor collects new orders and renewal decisions in its computer files. On the established date, the vendor produces a printout or computer tape of orders that it sends to the publisher along with payment. A late payment by a vendor typically results in the library missing the first or second issue of the next expected volume. Examples of missed issues due to late payment should be brought to the attention of the vendor account representative and, preferably, to the vendor representative responsible for scheduling publisher payments.

Smaller commercial publishers and some society publishers may not have the ability to process orders from vendors electronically and may therefore require orders and payment earlier to assure continuous subscriptions. Generally speaking, however, uninterrupted subscriptions can be assured if the library notifies its vendor of renewal and cancellation decisions by mid-October.

Cancellations

Once a cancellation decision has been made, it should be recorded in the check-in or payment record, specifying exactly when the cancellation takes effect. Most scholarly publications can only be cancelled at the end of the normal subscription period, and refunds of subscription payments are unusual. Cancellation decisions usually are reported to the vendor as a part of the annual renewal process or are forwarded directly to publishers for titles not ordered through a vendor. In the former case, cancellations should be carefully and clearly annotated on the renewal listing, and the cover letter to the vendor should list the cancelled titles.

Titles that have been cancelled may continue to arrive at the library for the first few months of the new subscription period. It is not necessary to return these issues to the publisher or vendor, and doing so may create unnecessary confusion for all concerned. Of greater use to the publisher is a brief letter indicating the library's reasons for the cancellation.

Payment Processing

Scheduling Payment

Exactly how and when the library processes subscription invoices may be dictated by the parent institution the library serves. However, in the case of payments to vendors, the cost of a library's subscriptions can be substantially affected by the vendor's payment terms. For this reason it is important to have a clear understanding of vendor payment options and how they can benefit the library.

Most serials vendors offer libraries financial incentives to make early payment for the coming year's subscriptions. The early payment does not commit the library to any specific renewals, and the library subsequently performs the normal renewal and cancellation notification process with the vendor. By making an early payment, however, the library earns a credit on its account that increases the amount of money available to pay its invoices. Vendors typically offer early payment credits as some percentage of the amount paid. A maximum credit is typically applied to payments received by the vendor prior to April 30, with the percentage falling thereafter to the point, usually in September or October, when no special credit is earned.

The early payment invoice usually is a one-line invoice based on projected subscription expenditures for the next year, but it can also be for a portion of the total amount. For example, if projected expenditures are $400,000 but the library only has $200,000 available for early payment, it can earn an early payment credit on that amount. Figure 3-7 illustrates a vendor statement showing an early payment and a credit on a library account, with invoices deducted from the account balance.

Some institutions may not permit early payments, but if the institution will allow them, the library should carefully weigh the advantages and disadvantages. There is an obvious financial benefit to the library by extending the buying power of its serials budget. Also, making a single early payment may eliminate the need for the library and the institution to process numerous individual invoices for payment, producing further savings to the institution. On the other hand, early payments to vendors represent a calculated risk, since it may be impossible to retrieve the funds if the library subsequently loses faith in the vendor or suffers an unexpected budget cut. Furthermore, for libraries that receive their funding based on a percentage increase over the previous year's expenditures, there may be no lasting benefit to the collection by garnering early payment credits.

Reviewing and Posting Invoices

Most automated serials systems have options for downloading vendor invoice information into the library's individual title payment records through magnetic tape or a diskette supplied by the vendor. Recently vendors have also begun distributing this data by file transfer over the Internet. In a manual system the invoice information is added by hand to the payment history for each title. In either case, essential elements of the invoice entry include the invoice number, invoice date, amount charged, and the volumes or chronological subscription term covered by the payment.

Regardless of how the information is recorded, invoices need to be carefully reviewed to be sure they represent the library's expectations. Each item on the invoice is compared with the order file to determine that it represents a title the library has ordered. It also may be necessary to question why certain titles are missing from the invoice. The correct number of copies is confirmed for each title, and the library notes what years and volumes are being invoiced to be certain these have not been paid already. Discrepancies should be documented and the vendor or publisher notified promptly.

The current price of each title on the invoice should also be compared with the previous amount paid for it. Staff conducting the review may be given guidelines for what is considered an acceptable percentage increase.

```
H A R R A S S O W I T Z
Booksellers & Subscription Agents
PO Box 2929 * 65019 Wiesbaden, Germany
```

STATEMENT OF ACCOUNT FOR EARLY ANUAL PAYMENT   PAGE ____
DATE: 06DEC94

HEALTH SCIENCES LIBRARY   CUSTOMER CODE: XXXXX-XXX
UNIVERSITY OF NORTH AMERICA
1142 ACADEMIC STREET   CUSTOMER NO: 9999999
MIDDLETOWN, IA 54621

ALL AMOUNTS IN US DOLLARS

DATE	TRANSACTION	NUMBER	ACCOUNT	CREDITS	DEBITS	BALANCE
17JUL94	EARLY PAYMENT	INV 1192	XXXXXXX	545,000.00		545,000.00
17JUL94	CREDIT FOR EARLY PAYMENT		XXXXXXX	21,800.00		566,000.00
26AUG94	DEDUCTION	INV 1572	XXXXXXX		326,427.48	239,572.52
20OCT94	PAYMENT ADD EARLY PYMNT FOR TRANSFERS	INV 1445	XXXXXXX	30,000.00		269,572.52
20OCT94	CREDIT FOR ADD EARLY PYMNT		XXXXXXX	600.00		270,172.52
05NOV94	DEDUCTION	INV 2203	XXXXXXX		239,768.83	30,403.69
06DEC94	CREDIT (CANCELLATIONS)	CR 41522	XXXXXXX	571.70		30,975.39
10DEC94	DEDUCTION	INV 257041	XXXXXXX		13,476.30	17,499.09
11FEB95	DEDUCTION	INV 270729	XXXXXXX		6,50.51	10,997.58
20APR95	DEDUCTION	INV 301777	XXXXXXX		8,462.34	2,535.24
TOTALS				597,971.70	594,636.46	2,535.24

Figure 3-7: Vendor Statement Showing Invoice Charges Applied Against Early Payment and Early Payment Credit (Courtesy of Otto Harrasowitz Booksellers and Subscription Agents, Wiesbaden, Germany)

For example, increases in excess of 20% might be flagged for higher level review. Extreme increases in the price of a journal usually represent an increase in frequency of publication. Nevertheless, sudden dramatic increases in the price of a title may initiate reconsideration of its benefit compared to its cost to the library. Invoice review also includes a review of the service charges applied, to ensure that the charges are in line with the terms agreed upon between the vendor and the library.

Price information can be a source of misunderstanding, and for this reason the library should clarify with the vendor exactly what prices are being used in various circumstances. Prices on invoices usually reflect the publisher's latest announced price for the current subscription year. Annual renewal invoices generated during the last few months of the year may partially or completely reflect prices established for the coming year. Vendors have recently initiated the helpful practice of noting on the renewal invoice whether the price is "firm" or not, thus indicating to the library whether or not additional charges should be expected. A less encouraging development is the trend for more and more publishers to charge substantially higher rates to institutional subscribers than they do to individuals.

Prices of foreign journals can be further complicated by currency exchange rates. Fortunately there is a trend for foreign publishers to establish an official U.S. dollar price for North American subscriptions, with the result that once they announce a price, it is uniformly charged by all vendors. If a foreign journal's price is established only in the local currency, the vendor usually converts this to a dollar price at the time that the invoice is generated. Fluctuations in international currency exchange rates can occasionally result in a vendor issuing either credits or added charge invoices for titles already billed and paid.

Management Issues

Budget Projections

The challenge of fiscal planning and budgeting is perhaps the most complex aspect of serials management, since only one fact can be certain about journal prices in the 1990s, and that is that they will increase each year. Two annual studies can be helpful, however, in identifying general trends in periodical prices for budgeting purposes. *Library Journal* annually publishes its periodical price index covering domestic and foreign publications [19], and *American Libraries* publishes the annual U. S. periodical price index, which may be more useful to small libraries with primarily domestic subscriptions [20].

Serials vendors also issue price projections beginning early in the calendar year and update these projections periodically as pricing information is released by publishers. Some of these projections are based on the type of library and on the mix of domestic and foreign titles. The projections are routinely distributed to the vendors' clients and frequently are summarized in the *Newsletter on Serials Pricing Issues* [21].

Individual library collections are unique, however, and they may not conform to the trends of the annual surveys. In addition, libraries frequently need to submit a budget request before these annual studies are published. Therefore, an internal analysis of the library's own expenditure trends should also be conducted. Since most serials expenditures are made in the fall, a good estimate of total annual expenditures can usually be made early in the calendar year.

Customized reports from vendors about the library's subscription costs can also assist in budgeting for serials. These reports usually can be supplied within a few days of their request. A most useful report for budgeting purposes shows the library's annual costs for each subscription for the past three years, so that long-term trends become apparent. Careful review of vendor reports and direct consultations with the vendor can assist the librarian in making realistic projections of future expenditures.

The number of foreign subscriptions in the collection can significantly affect budget projections due to the effects of currency exchange rates. Vendor reports can usually be arranged by country of publication to provide a profile of subscriptions affected by the various currencies. Based on such an analysis, periodic monitoring of the dollar exchange rate for the German mark and other foreign currencies can provide an early indication of cost trends to be anticipated.

Statistical Reporting

Parent institutions, accrediting bodies, and professional organizations routinely request statistics on the library's serials collection and expenditures. Commonly requested statistics include the following:

- Number of serial titles in the collection.

- Number of active serial titles in the collection.

- Number of paid subscriptions.

- Number of serial volumes in the collection.

- Number of serial volumes added annually.

- Annual expenditure for serials.

In addition, work flow statistics can be useful in monitoring the amount and complexity of work performed by staff. Common indicators of serials acquisitions work flow include the following:

- Number of new subscriptions placed.

- Number of items checked in.

- Number of claims entered.

- Number of invoice items posted.

Including data collection as a part of daily processes can be helpful in meeting requests from outside bodies for statistics about the library and for reviewing the work performed by the serials unit. Use of automated serials control systems can substantially reduce the number of statistics that need to be recorded manually.

Selection and Evaluation of Subscription Vendors

Selection of a New Vendor

The process used for selection of a vendor can be an informal one that results from personal discussions and verbal agreements or it can be the result of a formal bidding process ending in a negotiated contract. Institutional policy may require one approach or allow a range of options. A formal bid process focusing on the lowest service charge can be time-consuming if required on a repeated basis, and may not result in getting the best service for the library. A more balanced bid process, focusing on both costs and services, can provide the library with the opportunity to analyze and enumerate its requirements for a vendor and select the one that best meets its needs [22]. This is true both for libraries that are selecting a vendor for the first time and for libraries that are contemplating a switch from their current vendor.

Vendor proposals are generally based upon either a Request for Proposal (RFP) or Request for Quotation (RFQ) issued by the library. If the lowest possible service charge is the overriding factor in making the selection, then an RFQ may be more practical than an RFP. But if the overall service of the vendor is important to the library and the library is willing to pay a higher service charge to get the services it wants, then an RFP would be more useful. In either case, the library must provide a complete, up-to-date list of the current serials subscriptions for which it is seeking a vendor, so that the vendor understands the scope of the work and can calculate the service charge it will need to assess. Vendors typically quote their current prices for each of the titles listed, but such quotes should be considered with great caution as the basis for vendor comparisons. A lower price for a given title quoted by one vendor as compared to another can simply reflect the fact that one vendor has less current pricing information from the publisher than the other.

In the part of the RFP covering service specifications, a clear distinction should be made between mandatory requirements and desirable additional services. Sample documents obtained from colleagues at other libraries may provide a useful starting point for formulating this portion of the RFP. Vendors may also be willing to provide copies of RFPs they consider exemplary. In general, the RFP should itemize the services required by the library and should specify when and how the selection will be made. Many of the standards for evaluation of an existing vendor listed in the next section can be reframed as objective standards suitable for an RFP.

There are several ways of identifying prospective recipients of the RFP. *Library Journal* publishes an annual "Sourcebook" issue in December which includes the names and addresses of major full-service subscription agencies. The American Library Association also publishes an annotated directory of international subscription agents now in its sixth edition [23]. Most vendors exhibit at the major national and regional professional meetings where they distribute information about their services. Another important source of information on vendors is by word-of-mouth recommendations from experienced colleagues.

Vendors are accustomed to preparing responses to RFPs and usually can do so within six to eight weeks. While vendors are accustomed to this activity, the time and effort required to prepare responses is considerable. Each response therefore deserves thorough and thoughtful consideration by the library. When all responses are received, the replies of each vendor to each item in the RFP can be scored and tabulated for comparison. This comparison should provide an objective basis for selection of the vendor.

When comparing vendor proposals it is important to understand how the proposed service charge will be computed and applied. If service charges are assessed on a title-by-title basis, the library should ascertain whether there is a cap on the service charge for expensive titles and whether there is a minimum dollar amount charged for inexpensive titles. In addition, the library should determine if special orders, such as mid-year new title orders or backfile orders, will be assessed a higher service charge. Since overall service charges are usually based on the percentage of titles for which the publisher offers the vendor a substantial discount (a practice especially typical of the European STM publishers), libraries can usually negotiate lower overall service charges if they can add more foreign STM titles to the account.

Evaluation of a Current Vendor

Even for libraries that are basically satisfied with the service of their current subscription vendor, a periodic, formal evaluation of the vendor's service can be useful in enhancing the value of the library-vendor relationship. The ALA's *Guide to Performance Evaluation of Library Materials Vendors* can serve as a basic source for areas of evaluation, although it does not address serials vendors in detail [24].

Some specific benefits the library can expect to realize by undertaking a formal evaluation of its current subscription vendor are

Improved Vendor Performance

If the library is dissatisfied with the performance of a vendor, an attempt should be made to identify an objective basis for the dissatisfaction, and thereby establish mutually understood criteria for improved vendor performance.

Improved Library Procedures

A more thorough knowledge of vendor and library practices can result in improved library operations and efficiencies in serials acquisitions practices. For example, an evaluation may identify a duplication of effort between the library and the vendor that can be eliminated. The library may also be able to identify circumstances in which it is more effective to communicate directly with publishers, rather than through the vendor.

Lower Costs

Service charges are negotiable, and the library may be able to identify vendor services that it can do without or changes it can make to the mix of titles in the account to receive a more favorable service charge.

Elements of Vendor Evaluation

Specific methods for evaluating vendors vary based on the resources available in the library and the library's service priorities. Criteria which can be observed and documented, and examples of appropriate questions to consider follow [25].

Order Placement

The library should be able to expect that its orders will be accurately and promptly placed by the vendor and the that vendor will have the resources to handle the library's orders. Are orders placed and confirmed promptly? Are orders filled accurately? Can the vendor identify uncommon or new publishers without assistance from the library? Can orders be submitted in a variety of formats? How often does the library need to claim unfilled orders?

Annual Renewal of Subscriptions

Provided the library meets the vendor's timetable for submitting renewal orders and payments, it should expect continuous supply of its subscriptions. Does the annual renewal invoice correctly reflect the library's current subscriptions, including recent new title orders and cancellations? Are publishers receiving renewals and payments from the vendor in time to avoid lapsed subscriptions and missed January issues.

Dispatch Information

Publishers often notify vendors of delayed publications and issues published out of sequence, and this information should be relayed to the library by the vendor in a newsletter or a special report. Are dispatch notifications to the library sent soon enough to avoid unnecessary claims? Is there evidence that the vendor exerts its influence to encourage reliable deliveries from publishers?

Handling Claims

If the library uses more than one vendor, statistics on claims entered and claims filled by each vendor can be examined to determine if there is a reasonable explanation for variations in performance. Claim statistics can be compared with a comparable library to determine if the library is claiming more or less, and to indicate the relative effectiveness of the library's and vendor's claiming practices. The way in which a vendor processes claims can affect the need for second and third claims and can affect the library's operations. Are claims forwarded to the publisher without preliminary review, or are they compared to publisher dispatch reports and other publisher announcements to filter unnecessary claims? Does the vendor verify the library's order and payment for the title before sending a claim to a publisher?

Two quantitative measures of claiming performance include the calculation of the claim response rate and the claim success rate. The *claim response rate* is the ratio of the number of claims entered to the number of claims for which some response (even that it was placed after the publisher's deadline) is received. The *claim success rate* is the ratio of the number of claims entered to the number of claims fulfilled by receipt of the item claimed. The library can use these calculations as the basis for exploring with the vendor ways for improving claiming operations.

Replacements, Backfiles, and Sample Issues

Vendors can usually supply replacement and backfile orders either through publishers or through specialized back issue dealers. The library should review the frequency with which such orders cannot be supplied by the vendor. The review can identify situations in which ordering directly from the publisher is more advantageous to the library in terms of cost and speed of fulfillment. Similarly, if the library uses more than one vendor, a comparison of each vendor's performance in supplying replacement and backfile orders can serve as a basis for placing orders with the more successful vendor.

Vendors communicate regularly with publishers and can transmit sample issue requests for the library. Does the vendor accept sample requests in a variety of formats, e.g., by telephone, electronic mail, or letter? How promptly are samples received after being requested?

Condition of Material Received

Some vendors provide a reshipping service, usually for foreign titles. The vendor receives the issues, checks for missing items, consolidates them into batches, and ships them on a regular schedule to the library. In such cases, the vendor has control over the shipping conditions, and the library should expect material to arrive regularly, complete, and undamaged. During a selected evaluation period, shipment receipt dates can be noted to determine whether the expected delivery schedule is still being met, and any problems with the physical condition or completeness of the shipments should be noted. In some cases photographs may help document unacceptable packing or shipping conditions.

Cancellations

It is important to have a clear understanding of the vendor's cancellation policy. Are there added charges for canceling a subscription, and if so how are they assessed? What are the vendor's deadlines on cancellations? Does the vendor automatically request a refund for a canceled subscription if one is possible? Are cancellations noted as such on the next renewal listing? Are cancellations acknowledged promptly?

Invoices

Institutional needs and the library's automated serials control system may require some variations in the vendor's standard invoicing formats and procedures. The vendor's ability to comply with the library's specific needs for invoicing should be reviewed regularly. Is the timing of the annual renewal invoice flexible enough to meet library and institutional needs? Does the vendor provide ways to minimize the number of supplemental or bill-later invoices that need to be handled? Can the vendor produce an electronic version of the invoice to meet automated system specifications? Can electronic invoicing information be provided in formats that are compatible with standard database and spreadsheet software?

Prices

A method of evaluating the vendor's pricing practice is to compare prices on vendor invoices with the prices indicated in the issues or in the publishers' catalogs. This review can be done with a random sample of the subscription list or with all subscriptions from a few representative publishers. The objective is to identify discrepancies and to determine if they can be explained.

Service Charge

On a selected sample of invoices, the library can compute the assessed service charge as a percentage of the amount billed and compare this with the vendor's stated service charge. If the library has more than one account with the vendor and the accounts are assessed different service charges, it is especially important to review the accuracy of service charge assessments on invoices.

Reports

Most vendors offer an extensive range of customized statistical and financial reports, as well as reports intended to support analysis and evaluation of the serials collection. The library should specify the reports it needs and discuss these with the vendor. Most vendors are willing to develop new reports based on the needs of their customers. Are existing vendor reports sufficient to meet the library's needs? Are reports available in print and electronic formats? What is the turnaround time for receiving customized reports? For reports that include price projections, what is the vendor's track record for accuracy?

Selection and Evaluation of an Automated Serials Control System

Given the importance of serials in health sciences libraries, the quality of serials control functionality may be the deciding factor in selecting an integrated library system. Alternatively, libraries may opt for a stand-alone solution to their serials automation needs. In either case, the system must meet the needs of library staff and users for current and accurate information about the library's serials collection and the needs of library administrators for related management and financial information. An automated system should provide the library with opportunities for increased efficiencies in work flow and in staff assignments, and it should allow the library a broad range of options for configuring the system to meet the needs of its unique setting. Health sciences libraries have some unique system requirements that must also be considered, including support of National Library of Medicine subject headings, classification, journal title abbreviations, and SERLINE title numbers.

In evaluating potential automated systems the library should determine the extent to which they adhere to existing national standards. Relevant current standards include those for bibliographic information, holdings information, and electronic data interchange (EDI) for invoicing information. Additional standards for electronic data interchange of claims, responses to claims, and dispatch information are in development and should be included in systems as they are adopted. Current information on EDI standards for serials can be accessed conveniently through the Faxon Home Page (http://www.faxon.com).

Criteria to consider in selection and evaluation of automated serials control systems are outlined in the following lists. These lists are not exhaustive, but attempt to identify major functional requirements for effective serials management in a health sciences library. Over time these capabilities probably will be incorporated into most systems, and new capabilities will be needed. Libraries planning for their first or second generation system should consult lists of desirable features regularly published in *Library Technology Reports* and elsewhere in the library literature [26]. Specifications used by other libraries that have recently installed a new system are also useful, as is personal consultation with these libraries about their experiences in moving to the new system.

Public Search and Display

- The system supports record retrieval by journal title, journal title abbreviation, ISSN, and title or subject keyword, including use of Boolean operators.

- Searching can be limited to serials only.

- Holdings and receipt information for each copy of a selected title can be displayed.

- All individual issue receipts for a selected title can be displayed.

- Display of receipts can be limited to a selected year or volume.

- Serials item display includes circulation status, location, and notes.

Order Entry and Payment Processing

- The system accommodates the following types of procurement: subscriptions, standing orders, memberships, deposit accounts, gratis subscriptions, and donations.

- The system permits order entry using bibliographic records downloaded from bibliographic utilities and vendor files.

- On-order records are visible in public displays.

- The library has the ability to selectively suppress on-order records from public displays.

- The system produces printed and electronic purchase orders and cancellation notices.

- The system supports entry of invoice information by keyboard entry, tape load, and file transfer.

- The system accommodates entry of multiple invoice and credit transactions for a title in the same fiscal year, and cumulates total expenses for a title during a fiscal year.

- The system provides payment records at the copy level.

- Payment entries accommodate: invoice number, invoice date, vendor, transaction type (e.g., payment, credit, adjustment), volume(s), period of subscription, amount of transaction, fund charged or credited, date transaction posted, vendor comments, and library comments.

- The system allows review of all transactions on a selected invoice.

- The system allows review of all transactions for a selected title.

- The system allows review of all transactions with a selected fund code.

- The system automatically supplies default fund codes.

- The system supports output of invoice information to standard microcomputer database and spreadsheet programs.

Check-in

- The system provides predictive check-in functions, based on frequency and pattern of publication and the previously received issue.

- For purposes of prediction, the system accommodates a wide range of standard frequencies (including daily, weekly, biweekly, monthly, bimonthly, quarterly, biannual, annual, and biennial) and permits customized patterning of titles with nonstandard publishing schedules.

- The system allows easy editing of frequency and publication pattern within the check-in function.

- The system supports multiple levels of issue enumeration, including series, volume, issue, part, subpart, and supplement.

- The system allows check-in of the predicted issue with a single keystroke.

- The check-in record includes fields for special check-in instructions, retention notes, routing instructions, and dispatch information from the vendor.

- The system allows convenient check-in of an issue other than the predicted issue.

- The system allows check-in of multiple copies of a title, either individually or as a group.

- The system allows check-in of combined issues and special issues, such as supplements and separately published indexes.

- The system maintains check-in records in correct enumeration order even if they are received out of sequence.

- The system supports convenient creation of copy records, including bar code assignment, during check-in.

- The operator can view payment information from within the check-in function by a simple keystroke sequence.

- The system supports use of the SISAC bar code for check-in.

Claiming

- The system identifies at check-in when an issue has been skipped and flags it for claiming.

- The system identifies overdue issues and flags the records for review.

- The system alerts the operator when claimed items are checked-in.

- The system cancels further claims upon check-in of a claimed item.

- The system provides variable grace periods for late issues.

- The system permits the operator to delete a system-identified claim or to "force" a claim not identified by the system.

- The system allows production of a list of overdue issues for review.

- Claim records accommodate comments to the vendor regarding individual claims.

- Check-in records accommodate entry of vendor responses to individual claims.

- The system supports online transmission of claims to vendors and of claims responses to the library.

- The system generates second and third claims at library-defined intervals.

Report Production

- The library has the ability to produce financial, statistical, and descriptive reports at library-defined intervals and on demand, formatted according to library-defined specification.

- Routine reports include new title lists and counts, ceased and cancelled title lists and counts, current encumbrances, and fund balances.

- Cumulative statistical reports provide the number of active and inactive titles, the number of titles by source, by fund, and by frequency, and the number of issues checked-in and claimed during library-defined intervals.

- Expenditure reports permit analysis of expenditures by fund, by vendor, and by country of publication.

- The system can output statistical and management reports in formats compatible with standard microcomputer programs.

- The system includes an easy-to-use report generator for production of customized reports.

- The report generator permits filtering by, and output of, all fields in the serials acquisitions records.

- The system allows easy access to archived data.

- The system can output bibliographic and holdings data in MARC format and in other library-defined formats.

Emerging Issues in Serials Acquisitions

Developments during the next decade will significantly change the face of the serials marketplace and of serials-related procedures in libraries. It is likely, for instance, that the mergers and consolidation of serials vendors in the 1980s and early 1990s will continue to the point where there are only a few major subscription agents on each continent. With the increasing determination of libraries to restrain growth in overall serials cost and the increasing demands on vendors to implement sophisticated automated systems, fewer and fewer vendors will survive in the marketplace. Also, the increasing cost of getting established in the subscription business makes it doubtful there will be new participants in the foreseeable future. This trend suggests a growing need for librarians to understand and effectively use negotiating skills to maintain advantageous vendor agreements.

The potential of electronic data interchange for facilitating serials acquisitions activities will become clearer within the next few years. The promise of EDI and the ANSI X12 standard for electronic data interchange is currently being explored for a wide range of applications, including order entry, invoicing, claims, claim responses, and communication of publisher dispatch data. The major ILS vendors are all working on development of EDI-compatible systems. However, issues of expense and related telecommunications requirements may substantially delay widespread implementation.

The trend away from centralized computing toward a client/server environment of distributed databases suggests that library automation systems of the future may be very different from the systems common in the 1980s and 1990s. In the future it may be cheaper to discard old software and equipment than it is to upgrade them. This suggests the importance of maintaining automated serials records in standard formats that can be easily exported from one system to another.

Negotiating and monitoring license agreements will become an added responsibility of serials acquisitions. The requirement of license agreements as part of the acquisitions process is already common for CD-ROM and computer software purchases; the trend shows signs of spreading to printed products as well. For example, since 1992 the AMA has required a signed license agreement with explicit usage restrictions in order to obtain its printed membership directory, and in 1994 Gordon and Breach implemented a multilevel subscription pricing structure tied to specific library usage restrictions. License restrictions for electronic serials may increasingly carry similar restrictions and will need to be examined carefully to determine if and how the library can comply with them.

Hybrid print and digital serials are now commonly encountered, with the result that it has become increasingly difficult to separate the purchase of printed journals from the licensing of related digital products. Many electronic indexes already have varying prices based on the purchase of all or part of a related print product. Electronic supplements to print publications are becoming more common, and electronic journals with print supplements may be expected to follow the trend. All of these developments suggest that the library's serials acquisitions staff will need to become as knowledgeable about computer networks as they are about subscription prices.

Refinements in document supply systems are also blurring the line between title-level acquisitions (i.e. journal subscriptions) and article-level acquisitions. It may become easy and desirable to acquire only designated articles from a journal title, rather than order a full year subscription. This development will provide serious challenges to traditional methods of ordering, receiving, and managing the serials collection.

The death of the traditional printed journal still appears to be some decades away, but important experiments are already well underway to find a viable electronic alternative. It seems reasonable to predict that by the end of this decade, the electronic serial will be rewriting the rules for how libraries acquire and provide access to biomedical information.

References

1. Annual statistics of medical school libraries in the United States & Canada. 17th ed. Seattle, WA: Association of Academic Health Science Library Directors, 1995.

2. Basch NB, McQueen J. Buying serials: a how-to-do-it manual for librarians. New York: Neal-Schuman, 1990.

3. Dow SL. A selective directory of government document dealers, jobbers and subscription agents. Ser Libr 1988;14(1/2):157-86.

4. Afes VB, Wrynn PE. Biomedical journal title changes: reasons, trends, and impact. Bull Med Libr Assoc 1993 Jan;81(1):48-53.

5. Hepfer C. Serials pricing: the impact of exchange rates and currency trends. Ser Libr 1988;15(3/4):141-3.

6. Caelleigh AS. Journal supplements, libraries and the FDA. Bull Med Libr Assoc 1993 Apr;81(2):237-9.

7. Barry J, Griffiths J-M, Lundeen G. Automated system marketplace 1995, the changing face of automation. Libr J 1995 Apr 1;120(6):44-54.

8. Annual survey of automated library system vendors: integrated, multi-user, multifunction systems running on mainframes, minis, and micros that use a multi-user operating system. Libr Syst Newslett 1994 Mar/Apr;14(3/4):17-30.

9. Boss RW. Serials control in libraries: automated options. Libr Technol Rep 1984 Mar/Apr;20(2):89-281.

10. Boss RW. Serials control. Libr Technol Rep 1992 Jan/Feb;28(1):41-56.

11. Matthews JR, Parker MR. Microcomputer-based automated library systems: new series, part 1 . Libr Technol Rep 1993 Mar/Apr;29(2)147-302.

12. Matthews JR. Parker MR. Microcomputer-based automated library systems: new series, part 2 . Libr Technol Rep 1993 May/Jun;29(3)307-452.

13. Saffady W: Integrated library systems for minicomputers and mainframes: a vendor study, part I. Libr Technol Rep 1994 Jan/Feb;30(1):5-150.

14. Saffady W: Integrated library systems for minicomputers and mainframes: a vendor study, part II. Libr Technol Rep 1994;Mar/Apr; 30(2):155-323.

15. American Library Association. Association for Library Collections and Technical Services. Serials Section. Acquisitions Committee. Guidelines for handling library orders for serials and periodicals. Rev. ed. Chicago: American Library Association, 1992.

16. McKay SK, Piazza CJ. EDI and X12: what, why, who. Ser Rev 1992;18(4):7-10.

17. Miller JK, Peay W. Serials control and special problems. In: Darling L, Colaianni LA, Bishop D, eds. Handbook of medical library practice. 4th ed. v. 2. Chicago: Medical Library Association,1988:309-42.

18. Smith KR. Serials agents/serials librarians. Libr Res Tech Serv 1970 Winter;14(1):5-18.

19. Ketcham L, Born K. Serials vs. the dollar dilemma: currency swings and rising costs play havoc with prices: 35th annual report, periodical price survey 1995. Libr J 1995 April 15;120(7):43-49.

20. Alexander AW, Carpenter KH. U.S. periodical price index for 1995. Am Libr 1995 May 1;26(5):446-454.

21. Tuttle M, ed. Newsletter on serials pricing issues. listserv@unc.edu:subscribe prices [name].

22. Keating LR, Rogers MH. To bid or not to bid: is it still a choice? Ser Libr 1990;17(3/4):175-178.

23. Wilkas LR. International subscription agents. 6th ed. Chicago: American Library Association, 1994.

24. American Library Association. Collection Management and Development Committee. Guide to performance evaluation of library materials vendors. Chicago: American Library Association, 1988.

25. American Library Association. Association for Library Collections and Technical Services. Serials Section, Acquisitions Committee. Guide to performance evaluation of serials vendors, Draft 5, December 1992.

26. Boss RW. Technical services functionality in integrated library systems. Libr Technol Rep 1992 Jan/Feb:28(1):1-109.

4

Serials Management Issues

Barbara A. Carlson

Like the format itself, serials management has undergone a tremendous transformation in recent decades due to the proliferation of serial literature, inadequate library budgets, advanced publishing technologies, library automation, and the rising expectations of library users. Its complexity derives from the need to blend efficient internal technical operations with the service needs of the community of library users and, at the same time, to keep an eye on emerging trends and developments in the serials publishing industry. Balancing these diverse imperatives constitutes the challenge that serials librarians face.

With journals the format of choice for the medical scholarly record, health sciences library serials collections and their related services provide especially fertile ground for library innovation today. Opportunities to stretch traditional library roles abound in the ways libraries control and provide access to this literature. Electronic delivery of scholarly information during the next decade will further change the roles of libraries, subscription agencies, and publishers.

As automation facilitates the integration of many library functions, serials management decisions continue to be at the crossroads of technical and public services. Collection development, acquisitions, cataloging, interlibrary loan, document delivery, circulation, reference, and automated systems planning—all directly impact serials operations and vice versa. Serials collections have always challenged libraries with complex management issues, but never has there been such turmoil as during this transitional period from print to electronic scholarly communication. Traditional values, assumptions, organizations, formats and structures are being simultaneously reexamined and reconfigured within the library-vendor-publisher-scholar domain. Much of today's professional wisdom may have little relevance for the challenges of tomorrow.

One of the reasons that serials management interconnects with other library functions is that serials titles and the items themselves continue to cycle through internal processes during the life of the serial. Unlike monographs that are ordered, cataloged, processed, and moved on to library shelves and users in a one-time operation, serials are ordered, cataloged, stored, and inventoried in a recurring way throughout the life of the title. Simply put, serials revisit.

This chapter will explore the processes that lie beyond the primary acquisition activities of ordering, check-in, and claiming. These processes and issues include the following:

- Physical arrangement and labeling.

- Disposition of duplicates and exchange management.

- Binding and repair.

- Holdings record creation and maintenance.

- Union listing.

- Special services provided directly to users.

Upon first glance, it is tempting to suggest that not much has changed over the last decade in some of these areas, but a closer look reveals that changes have filtered deeply into these processes.

Automation and the Library User

Perhaps the most significant factor transforming the way serials are managed in libraries is the fact that automated systems are making serials processing records, or information derived from them, directly accessible to local and remote users and staff members. The potential usefulness of this information is obvious, given the fact that questions concerning periodicals and holdings continue to constitute the single largest category of questions asked in biomedical libraries [1]. Whether this wealth of newly available information actually contributes to users' success in locating library material is an area ripe for study; whether public services staff members are correctly interpreting such information is unmeasured as well. What does seem clear is that serials management decisions, especially in an automated environment, have a direct effect on the success or failure of the library's collection-based services [2-3]. In any event, automation has undeniably brought a greater public dimension to the tasks of serials management.

The level of detail, accuracy, timeliness, clarity, and consistency with which records are created and maintained has an immediate impact on the level of library service that can be rendered. As serials change title, split, merge, die, revive, spawn sections, misnumber, change format, absorb each other, add or drop supplements, change publishers, change scope and purpose, become multimedia, and form companion publications, there is little wonder that the simple question, "Do you have this journal?" may not be easily answered without unraveling one or more mysteries. Couple these possibilities with changing status conditions, such as missing, at bindery, in repair, on loan, mutilated, claimed, and never received, and the odds seem hopelessly against the user finding what is needed, unless the library has a consistent and understandable system for communicating information about the serials collection to library users.

Historically, serials control was synonymous with multiple, single-purpose files; currently, consolidated, multipurpose files are both feasible and desirable. Serials record keeping has moved from having many separate staff-access files to comprehensive public-access systems that link bibliographic and holdings information to access and availability data. Automation has permitted the floodgates of serials data to open, creating new problems and dilemmas. At the same time, advances in electronic publishing technology, including CD-ROM and online journals, are placing new demands on the flexibility and speed of serials data management.

Physical Arrangement and Labeling

Much interest and energy has been devoted to increasing intellectual access to serials and their content, but physical ease of access is also an integral part of finding information within library collections. Additionally, physical arrangement impacts on the efficiency of internal operations such as bindery pickup, and can either mitigate or exacerbate the problem of locating missing issues. How a library arranges the serials collection may be the result of many factors: physical facility design, historic decision-making, assumptions about user-behavior, national library standards, library staff configurations, and compatibility with other libraries within the institution. Typical decisions involve choices between classified versus alphabetic arrangements, consolidated journal runs versus chronological splits, on-site versus remote storage for older volumes, and the pros and cons of separate shelving areas for the latest day's or week's receipts.

Alphabetical and Classified Arrangements

Health sciences libraries, both hospital and academic, as polled by the Public Service Division of the National Library of Medicine, reported that 79% of them arrange journal collections alphabetically by title [4]. This percentage is not surprising since health sciences collections are usually of small to moderate size, and the interdisciplinary nature of biomedical research reduces the usefulness of arrangements classified by subject.

Title arrangements are simple to understand for the user and generally do not require any special location labeling on the issues. However, when both an initialism and full form of the title appear on the cover, the title designated for shelving must be graphically identified. This identification is commonly done by underlining the first letters or words of the preferred title element, a process sometimes referred to as "hooking." For unbound journal issues, this is a simple matter. However, for some monographic series where the series title may not appear on either the cover or spine, a label with the filing title may need to be added. Some libraries routinely provide such title labels on all issues.

Title arrangement does bring with it the attendant problems of alphabetization. The library may favor word-by-word alphabetizing, or it can use keyword filing, in which prepositions and articles are ignored and acronymns are filed as words [5]. This method tends to aid users working from title abbreviations, since it forgives users for not knowing, for example, that Ann Rheum Dis actually stands for Annals of *the* Rheumatic Diseases. While such access benefits users, it sometimes makes technical processing operations problematic, since computer filing generally regards all words. Many medical libraries also shelve initialisms at the beginning of each letter, but again computer filing may not correlate with the shelf arrangement. Some large biomedical libraries, while basically following an alphabetic arrangement, use the NLM-assigned W1 classification number with a Cutter number to give titles an unambiguous location designation.

For title variations and preceding or successive titles, dummy volumes or signs can be used to direct users to the related titles. Similarly, markers can be placed to direct library users from variant forms of the title, such as initialisms, to the correct shelving title.

Chronological Divisions

In libraries that retain journal issues long enough to require binding, serials collections are typically split into a section for bound volumes and a section for display and browsing of current unbound issues. Very small collections may permit the integration of bound and unbound issues without sacrificing browsability. Additionally, bound journal collections in larger libraries often must be divided either alphabetically or chronologically and split between floors or building wings or a remote storage facility. A chronological split (e.g., pre-1980 and 1980+) has the potential advantage of concentrating the most heavily used portion of the collection in the most accessible area of the building. It has the disadvantage of possibly misleading some library users who are not aware of both shelving areas.

Current unbound journal collections are also subject to subdivision in libraries that provide a separate display area for the current day's or week's receipts. The usefulness of such current awareness displays must be weighed against the problems they cause for users attempting to locate specific issues and for staff facing additional processing tasks. In general, the greater the number of sublocations within the serials collection, the more complicated the user's task becomes in locating materials. To make such an arrangement truly useful as a current awareness aid, serials staff must be consistent about the time of day when issues are cycled on and off of the current receipts display. Also, issues removed for photocopying or reading must be redisplayed promptly.

Navigation Aids

No matter what physical arrangement is chosen, users still need clear signage and other navigational aids to assist them is negotiating the serials collection. At a workshop on improving physical access to serials collections, these ideas were suggested.

- Increase public service to periodicals, perhaps relocating the serials department so that it can be responsible for this function.

- Create a current issue reading room.

- Add building level and stack numbers to existing periodical holdings lists.

- Add more location notes to online catalogs.

- Use different colored classification labels to help library staff quickly move used materials back to the proper location and also help librarians explain to patrons which items are periodicals (usually noncirculating) and which are monographs [6].

Such suggestions are not prescriptive but serve as representative actions that librarians might consider in designing policies that strike the proper balance between serials collection management and user needs.

Labels, Bar Codes, and Security Strips

In addition to indicating the correct shelving location for each serial item either by "hooking" or adding a call number, physical processing of incoming serials also involves adding library ownership marks and strips or labels for theft detection systems. Some labeling, such as affixing permanent spine labels to prebound serials may be completed by the books processing staff. Although security concerns focus primarily on bound volumes, unbound issues may also be security labeled to deter users from unauthorized borrowing. Libraries with large collections may choose to selectively strip or label titles with a history of theft, since treating all issues can be expensive. Some binders may offer, as part of their services, insertion of such strips in volumes at the time of binding.

Automation has given rise to an additional processing step for many serials operations: bar coding. Local bar codes can be applied to allow for automated circulation, and to gather statistics on internal use and external circulation. As with the use of security strips or labels, the extent of local bar code application is determined by assessing the value of the resulting use measurement in relation to the time and effort required to affix and scan the labels. Some automated serials control systems provide efficient ways of "collapsing" the bar coded issue records and their associated use data after the issues are bound into a single volume.

Unsolicited Issues, Replacements, and Duplicates

One serials management problem that is not likely to disappear any time soon is the management and disposal of unwanted volumes and issues of journals, sometimes referred to generically as "duplicates." Literally tons of material each year finds its way to libraries as gifts from well-meaning donors, as unsolicited mailings by publishers, and as the result of errors by publishers, vendors, or libraries in the distribution and claiming process. As sources for filling gaps in the collection, such materials are welcomed additions, especially in times when fiscal restraints limit materials budgets. However, it is a misconception to suppose that this material comes without a price, since considerable staff time and space is required for screening and processing. The most troublesome material is that which the library does not need or want and yet costs the library time, space, and effort to redistribute or discard.

Medical libraries have a long history of finding creative ways to move the unwanted material to people and institutions that can use it. The primary methods of redistribution are duplicate exchanges, backfile dealers, and book sales or give-away programs. The other alternative for disposition, outright discard, should be viewed as a last resort. It is, however, employed by almost all libraries to some degree as a practical option under varying circumstances. No matter what the method of disposal, it is important to stamp the material "discarded" or "withdrawn," in order to forestall its rearrival at the library's doorstep. This particular type of serials "revisiting" is clearly undesirable and largely preventable.

Given adequate space and staff, duplicate and unsolicited journal issues can serve as valuable in-house sources for replacements of missing or mutilated issues or to fill user requests while volumes are at the bindery. Also, they can serve as review copies in the selection process for new subscriptions. There are other good reasons for holding onto apparently unsolicited or duplicate materials. Most importantly, issues that appear to be unsolicited may subsequently be identified as parts of a regular subscription continuing under a new title. Also, "duplicates" may turn out not to be duplicates at all, but rather the result of erroneous check-in records or issue misnumbering by the publisher. In any case, duplicates and unsolicited items have a limited shelf life before they become unwanted management burdens. Finding new homes for these publication orphans requires a variety of resources and strategies.

Medical Library Association Exchange

One of the first projects the Association of Medical Librarians undertook shortly after it was formed in 1898 was to organize a duplicate exchange of periodical issues among its member libraries [7]. The MLA Exchange, as it is known today, survives as a valuable if problematic organizational service. As a batching of individual lists of surplus serials items from participating libraries, its unwieldy paper format, which is both time-consuming to use and costly to produce and distribute, has been the source of frustration to librarians eager to redistribute resources. In 1995, MLA began making the exchange lists available in ASCII file format, which substantially enhances the ability of libraries to search the lists for specific titles. Ongoing attempts to contain costs, improve the product, and to further automate the process are continuing quests for the elusive exchange grail, spurred on by a long-standing spirit of interlibrary cooperation.

In 1991, the MLA Exchange Advisory Committee conducted a pilot project with over 200 MLA libraries in conjunction with ABACIS, Inc. and its software product SerialsQuest, which automatically matches available items with searches for wanted ones. Since this automated service did not meet the needs of all users of the Exchange, the paper version has been retained, with SerialsQuest serving as a nonsponsored option. Many medical libraries continued to use SerialsQuest after the pilot project ended and comprise a large portion of the database.

SerialsQuest and Other Library Serials Exchanges

With access to approximately 250,000 serials issues, the libraries that participate in SerialsQuest earn credits through trading issues and volumes and pay small fees for items they request. When matches are found, SerialsQuest sends the requesting library, by electronic mail or an automatic download to the library's fax machine, information on the match, giving the library the option to pursue the transaction. Since the pilot project, SerialsQuest has become a regular service of The Faxon Company, available to all libraries whether or not they are subscription account customers.

With the advent of listservs and electronic discussion lists on the Internet, librarians have used these as independent means of distributing lists of duplicate journals. An MLA-sponsored electronic exchange list using a listserv or some other Internet facility, is currently being considered as an MLANET component. In September 1994, the Readmore subscription agency announced BACKSERV, a listserv that provides a forum for listing both available and desired serials back issues and duplicates [8]. Because of the heavy concentration of medical titles on BACKSERV, a separate list (BackMed) was created for just these titles. In addition to these efforts at the national level, health science libraries participate in local, regional, and chapter exchanges. Hospital, government, and Area Health Education Center (AHEC) libraries are more likely to use these consortial arrangements than are academic health sciences libraries [9].

Foreign Distribution of Unwanted Journals

For material that is commonly held within the United States and difficult to exchange, health sciences libraries have been resourceful in finding grateful recipients overseas. Philanthropic groups send items to developing countries, often reimbursing or absorbing the costs of shipping. It is advisable to check directly with such donor groups before forwarding donations. Each group has its own requirements and procedures, may only deal with recent publications or bound volumes, or may not handle journal donations at all. A few noteworthy organizations are listed in Table 4-1 [10]. Donor libraries may need to offer a list of donations for review, house the material for a time while communicating with potential recipients, pay shipping charges, and pack the shipment according to set specifications. Libraries entering into cooperative distribution agreements must keep in mind that recipient libraries are not places to unload material indiscriminately. Much effort is necessary by the partners on both ends to make such arrangements work.

Local community service organizations, as well as local physician groups, may be contacted to determine if they are sponsoring donation projects. An extensive although now somewhat dated list of foreign exchanges and charities was compiled by Ellen R. Cooper [11]. Detailed information can be found in the *Manual for International Book and Journal Donations*, which is available from the American Council of Learned Societies, 228 East 45th Street, New York, NY 10017-3398 [12]. A general overview of supplying surplus medical journals and books from U.S. libraries to institutions in foreign countries is provided by Ruelle [13]. There are periodic postings on Internet discussion lists regarding special international needs, and a search of the lists' archives can supply additional leads.

Also, it is worth remembering that libraries struck by disasters often need donations. If material for rebuilding working collections is on hand, the donating library should contact the affected library to determine if the potential donations fit the disaster-struck library's needs and recovery plans. Pleas for such material are often posted on electronic bulletin boards or in regional publications.

Commercial Sources

Academic medical libraries are likely to offer their unwanted journals and to seek needed volumes by using commercial backfile dealers. Table 4-2 provides a list of some major dealers. The list is by no means exhaustive, and other specialized dealers that are regionally oriented might better suit the needs of a particular library, e.g., Antonio R. Raimo, specializing in dentistry journals, or Hawkeye Book and Magazine Company in Redfield, South Dakota. Librarians should investigate various services, their subject scope, terms for fulfillment, current rates for purchases, and quotes for donations, and then establish working relationships with the firms that provide the best services and arrangements suitable to the library's needs. As a general rule, back-volume dealers concentrate on the last five or ten years of high-demand journals [14]. The library, if allowed by its institution, may receive payment for items provided to dealers, or a credit toward the future purchase of material, depending on the company's terms and the library's needs and policies. Good sources of information about dealers are

Table 4-1: Examples of Organizations That Accept Journal Donations

Medical Books for China, International
13021 East Florence Avenue
Santa Fe Springs, CA 90670-4505
Telephone: 310-946-8774; (800) 554-2245
FAX: 310-946-0073

Books for Asia
The Asia Foundation
451 Sixth Street
San Francisco, CA 94119
Telephone: 415-982-4640 Ext. 243 or 230
FAX: 415-543-8131

The Brother's Brother Foundation
Education Program Coordinator
824 Grandview Avenue
Pittsburgh, PA 15211-1442
Telephone: 412-431-1600
FAX: 412-431-9116

International Book Project
1440 Delaware Avenue
Lexington, KY 40505
Telephone: 606-254-6771

---

the *Directory of Back Issue Dealers*, obtainable from the North American Serials Interest Group, (NASIG) [15], advertisements in library journals, and other librarians.

Some subscription agencies have special arrangements with backfile dealers. They may offer online access to the backfile dealer's stock through the subscription agency's electronic gateway, and may also maintain their own stock of duplicates. As an example, Readmore offers searchable access to the stock of Jerry Alper, Inc. and G. H. Arrow, Inc. as part of its online BACKSERV project. EBSCO's Missing Copy Bank contains very current issues that have been donated for redistribution, with a special emphasis on titles indexed in *Abridged Index Medicus*. There is no charge for requested items, but the database is somewhat limited in coverage. It is offered as an online service to EBSCO customers, who also have online access to Kraus Periodicals through EBSCONET. Faxon's SerialsQuest, as mentioned previously, offers automatic offline matching of wanted and needed items. Faxon, like some other commercial dealers, also provides a customized

Table 4-2: Examples of Commercial Backfile Dealers

Alfred Jaeger, Inc.
66 Austin Blvd.
Commack, NY 11725
Telephone: 516-543-1500; (800) 969-5247
FAX: 516-543-1537

J. S. Canner and Company, Inc.
10 Charles St.
Needham Heights, MA 02194-2906
Telephone: 617-449-9103
FAX: 617-449-1767

Jerry Alper, Inc.
271 Main St. P.O. Box 218
Eastchester, NY 10707
Telephone: 914-793-2100
FAX: 914-793-7811

G.H. Arrow Company
P.O. Box 676
Bala Cynwyd, PA 19004
Telephone: 215-227-3211; (800) 775-2776
FAX: 215-221-0631

Research Periodicals & Book Services, Inc.
11231 Richmond Ave.
Suite 106
P.O. Box 720728
Houston, TX 77272
Telephone: 713-556-0061; (800) 521-0061
FAX: 713-556-1406

Kraus Periodicals
358 Saw Mill River Road
Millwood, NY 10546-1035
Telephone: 914-762-2200; (800) 223-8323
FAX: 914-762-1195

Walter J. Johnson, Inc.
355 Chestnut Street
Norwood, NJ 07648
Telephone: 201-767-1303
FAX: 201-767-6717

search service for desired items, including contacting publishers, and a complete range of second-hand sources.

The United States Book Exchange (USBE) offers its exchange services to institutional, public, and corporate libraries from its stockpile of duplicates in a warehouse in Cleveland, Ohio. USBE handles both journal and book material, operates on a membership basis, and assesses modest handling charges for fulfillment. Member libraries are expected to make donations of materials regularly. A booklet that details USBE's activities and membership information is available from USBE, 2969 West 25th Street, Cleveland, OH 44113. Similar information is available at the USBE home page, http://www.usbe.com. USBE deals with libraries in developing countries and those of the former Soviet block that use USBE's donational program stock. Sometimes USBE assumes freight charges to aid in donations from U.S. libraries to needy non-U.S. libraries. As Garno reported on the first thirty-five years of USBE, the greatest demand has been for health sciences materials, with nearly 30 % (some four million) of the items placed being health related materials [16]. Today, over fifty years since its inception, USBE still plays an important role in redistributing medical publications.

In-house Disposition

To dispose of unwanted items including journals, libraries sometimes hold periodic in-house sales, although these efforts are mostly used to relocate items rather than to raise revenues. Libraries may also have permanent "give away" areas to allow patrons the benefit of library discards. Again, it is important to deprocess items completely by marking through identifying stamps and labels and using a discard stamp to guard against any misunderstanding of ownership in the future.

Binding

For most health sciences libraries, a binding program should be implemented that facilitates both collection use and preservation. Although the binding itself is generally contracted out to a commercial library binder, binding involves a substantial amount of in-house preshipment preparation and postshipment evaluation and processing. Basic components of the process are

- Selecting material for binding.

- Gathering and grouping items into new collective units.

- Preparing in-house records and lists.

- Preparing instructions for the binder.

- Packing and labeling the shipment.

- Receiving the returned shipment.

- Processing the bound volumes in preparation for reshelving.

- Returning the material to library shelves.

Libraries that retain only recent journal holdings or that systematically acquire serials in microform may find that the cost and internal effort of binding is not justified.

A library binding program is actually a microcosm that reflects the serials management program as a whole. It has a crucial impact on the library's service to users and is dependent on the success of other serials acquisition functions, such as accurate check-in and claiming. Proper administration of the program requires in-depth knowledge of binding structure, materials, and techniques; a thorough knowledge of serials publication behavior on a title-by-title basis; a full awareness of the special behavior and needs of the library's user groups; and a combination of business and communication skills.

Growing concerns for the preservation of library materials, changes in library binding standards, limited library budgets, and the introduction of automated systems have altered the essence of binding programs and shifted many decisions and responsibilities from binders to library staff. Good binders continue to take the major responsibility for choosing the most effective methods of binding, but are receptive to those libraries that wish to become more active in the decision-making. Unfortunately, in spite of the increased opportunities and added options, binding is mistakenly viewed in some quarters as a routine and essentially clerical function. Its real importance in the preservation, order, and use of the collection is frequently underestimated.

Binding and Public Service

To users, binding is commonly seen as a barrier to access and an unnecessary evil. Many users searching the journal literature are oblivious to the reasons for and the process of binding, but quickly learn to blame all failures to locate journal materials, for whatever cause, on this mysterious process called "the bindery." To reduce user frustration and volume inaccessibility during the binding process, technical services and public services staff must cooperate to determine the use patterns of the library's patrons and set an appropriate time to bind. Judgments about when to bind high-use, high-frequency journals are the hardest to make. Integrating knowledge of course curricula and supporting resources with library planning can reduce user dissatisfaction and library failure in some instances. More difficult to accommodate are researchers whose patterns of use are more varied.

It has been the experience of some academic health sciences libraries that current awareness services, most notably *Current Contents*, create a peak demand for the journals they index at a predictable time [17](generally from zero to eight weeks after receipt), and a corresponding call from users of these services that bindery preparation be postponed until after that period. However, binding volumes immediately upon receipt of the first issue of the next bibliographic volume is a common binding procedure for libraries, especially those which use automated serials control systems that prompt for binding readiness. Although longer binding delays may be requested by some library users, an increase in lost or stolen issues is likely to be the result of allowing unbound issues to accumulate. Satisfactory solutions have yet to be found to this perplexing problem.

In biomedical libraries these decisions are especially difficult because information in recent journal issues can be so critical to patient care needs and to grant-funded research. Coordination with interlibrary loan and document delivery services can ameliorate the problem somewhat by providing alternative sources for materials that are at the bindery. Turn-around time for material at the bindery is a related concern for health sciences libraries, but most commercial binders require an average of three to four weeks. In any case a regular, preset schedule of pickups and deliveries can assist library users in planning around bindery periods.

Binding as a Preservation Strategy

Binding makes journal issues easier to locate, to shelve, to protect from damage and theft by users, and to preserve as information packages. As a comprehensive plan, library binding has been recognized as the cornerstone of collection preservation. Biomedical libraries, with the leadership of NLM's National Preservation Program for the Biomedical Literature, treat library binding of books, and journals in particular, as a major preservation activity [18]. In 1986, the NLM Preservation Section was established and became responsible for preservation education, disaster prevention and recovery, management of contracts for binding, and preservation microfilming, and for providing leadership and funding opportunities to the medical library community [19].

Individual library binding programs fall within this national framework and are guided by evolutionary changes in library binding industry standards as developed by binders, librarians, and suppliers of materials. Walker states that library binding may be viewed as a conservation measure if it extends the life of the book and if the option to rebind remains [20]. Whether or not this happens depends on many factors, and librarians have great influence over the outcome. With acid-free paper now being used by the majority of biomedical publishers, commercial library binding standards for binding techniques and materials can create information packages that represent a balance between current ease of use and long-term archival integrity.

Binding Standards

Since 1935 when the Library Binding Institute (LBI) was founded, there have been eight editions of the *Library Binding Institute Standard for Library Binding*, and a new standard that addresses materials, techniques, and performance measures is under development as a joint NISO/LBI undertaking [21]. These standards outline minimum requirements for bound volume construction in terms of technical and material specifications. Specifications are defined for suitable methods of page attachment; collation (i.e., checking for the arrangement and completeness of content); trimming, rounding, and backing of the textblock; attachment of the cover boards; spine stamping; and the quality of materials used for endpapers, binder boards, coverings, adhesives, and threads for sewn volumes. A glossary of binding terms also helps librarians and binders speak the same language.

Through the seventh edition (1981), the use of high quality materials and techniques to produce a strong, durable product was the driving principle [22]. The standard was known as "Class A," and it required, among other things, a strong but somewhat inflexible method of leaf attachment known as "oversewing." While increased levels of photocopying raised flexibility concerns about oversewn volumes, libraries still demanded affordable, quality bindings of sturdy construction. The focus increasingly turned to producing a product that could withstand the rigors of photocopying, remain economically affordable, and satisfy sound preservation principles.

The current eighth edition (1986) of the *Standard* backs away from the old Class A emphasis, embraces double-fan adhesive binding as an alternative to oversewing, and offers a wide array of options for both library and binder [23]. One related trend that has emerged has been the switch from "custom" periodical collation to "standard" periodical collation. Custom collation requires that the binder, in accordance with library specifications, rearrange the title page, table of contents, index, and supplements; remove the covers and advertisements; guarantee the order of issues within the volume; check for the inclusion of all issues; and provide page-by-page

checking for missing, misordered, or damaged pages. "Standard" periodical collation generally requires the binder to inspect only for the correct
issue order and overall completeness of the volume. Except for these two
requirements, standard collation generally means "bound as received." If
a library wishes the volume content rearranged in a special order, the
library establishes the volume order in its preparation work. Many medical
libraries now use standard collation for the majority of titles they bind, with
only a few titles receiving custom collation. In addition to the substantial
cost benefit of standard collation, some libraries also view the lack of
advertising removal and page rearrangement as a positive benefit in preserving the material as a matter of historic record.

The current LBI Standard, with its enhanced options for materials and
techniques, is a reaction to changing expectations and conditions. In many
ways, the current standard complicates the binding tasks for libraries, since
it provides libraries with more opportunities for binding decisions than
were accommodated by the Class A standard. As suggested in the *Guide to
the Library Binding Institute Standard for Library Binding*, libraries may choose
to inspect and send specific instructions with each volume, provide general
guidelines to the binder, or abdicate such decisions by relying on the
binder's personnel to make the decisions [24].

Preshipment and Postshipment Procedures

Libraries identify items to be collected for binding in various ways, e.g.,
by physical inspection of current journal shelves, by cues from the check-in
staff, by printed "pull" slips generated from an automated system, or by a
combination of these methods. Based on one or more of these cueing
sources, the library staff member gathers, examines, and groups issues in
a chronological and numeric order. It is important to coordinate bindery
gathering with check-in records to ensure that all issues and supplements
are picked up. Separately issued indexes can be especially troublesome
since they typically arrive well after the volume is otherwise complete and
can easily be overlooked. Some reasonable effort to include them in bound
volumes should be considered, as they provide index information at the
point of actual use and may help users untangle erroneous or incomplete
citations.

Periodicals are bound according to established specifications for cover
material and color, lettering type and position, and volume thickness.
Generally, physical volumes should not be more than two inches thick, and
titles produced on heavy, clay-coated paper should be bound in smaller
units. The library's role in preparing materials for binding has generally
been limited to issue gathering, filling out binding orders, and record-keeping prior to the pickup of the shipment by the binder. During the last decade

in some libraries, especially those accepting "standard" binding services from their commercial binder, the library staff has assumed additional responsibility for examining the condition and nature of the material and collating journal issues. According to Parisi, examination and collation consist of nine steps:

- Test paper for embrittlement.

- Check for missing issues or leaves.

- Check for proper sequence of issues and leaves.

- Check for and mend any damaged leaves.

- Move the title page, contents, and index to their proper places in the volume.

- Remove advertisements.

- Remove paper covers from serial issues.

- Determine the method of leaf attachment.

- Check margins and note instructions for trimming [25].

The level of commitment that a library makes to these activities is determined by the knowledge of its binding staff, the time allotted for such decisions, the library's financial resources, and agreements between the library and the binder.

Once the newly grouped units are gathered and collated, written instructions for each physical volume are created on binding slips. If the library does not use an automated binding system that can generate multipart slips, the binder should provide slips with preprinted, title-specific information produced from the binder's title database. Figure 4-1 shows a representative binding slip. One or more copies of each slip travel with the volume to the bindery, and one copy is retained by the library. Volumes are tied or banded with large rubberbands, and data are updated in all serials records. A final cross check of the tied units with the binding slips and a consolidated shipment list is advisable before boxing the shipment by format and desired treatment. Until the time when the shipment is packed, items should be made accessible to users for short periods of time upon request.

When the shipment is returned from the bindery, volumes are unpacked and arranged on work area shelves, where they are checked to determine if all volumes were returned. Missing volumes should be reported immediately to the binder. Because binders are not infallible, checking each volume against its binding slip for accuracy of spine lettering, cover color,

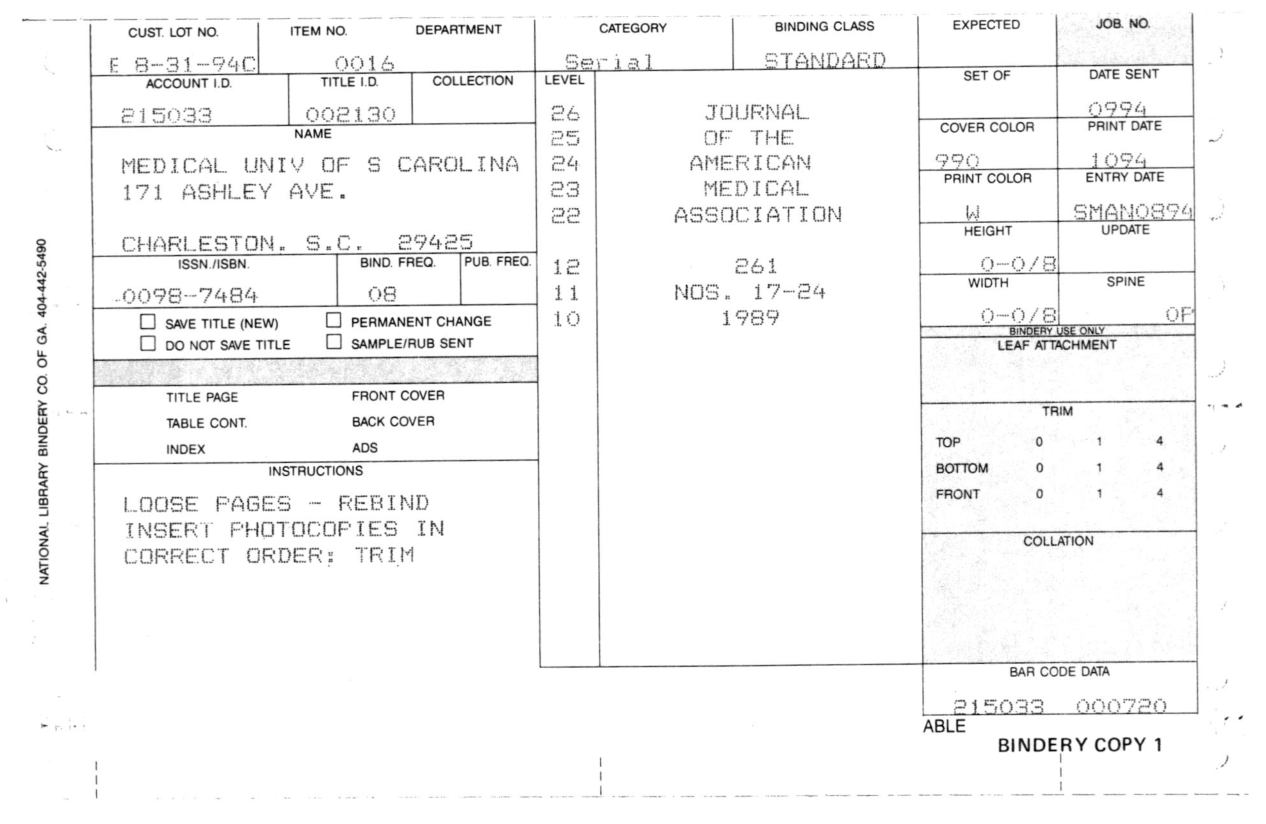

Figure 4-1: Binding Slip

and specific binding instructions is a useful exercise. When errors in spine lettering are discovered, library personnel must judge whether the error can be corrected in-house or should be sent back to the bindery, taking into consideration the severity of the error and the level of user-demand for the item. Quickly fanning through the volume to check the order of issues and for any trimming that may have damaged text or illustrations are useful precautions, although spot-checking volumes can suffice if the percentage of such mistakes runs at an acceptable level. Spot-checking for problems such as textblocks not squared in their cases, sloppy construction techniques, inferior materials, and inflexible hinge movement can also be valuable if the library is at all unsure of the binder's quality standards.

Once the volume passes inspection, marks of ownership are applied, a security strip and a date due slip may be affixed, and local bar codes attached for tracking circulation or in-house use. Binding and other serials records are updated to reflect the revised holdings of bound and unbound issues. When the binding invoice is received, the total number of volumes bound, the accuracy of the price-per-volume charge, and any extra charges should be reviewed.

Leaf Attachment Techniques

Although selecting what to bind has always been within the purview of the library, choosing a suitable method of leaf attachment for each book or journal volume is still primarily the binder's job [26]. As indicated previously, for many years "Class A" binding dictated a sewn binding for nearly all volumes. As publishers reduced the size of inner margins to maximize the number of words per page and cut their costs by using adhesive-bound construction for single issues, binders and librarians found that sewn bindings were not necessarily the best choice for every title and every library situation. Librarians and binders agreed to alter the standards to aid openability and allow for a range of leaf attachment options, including oversewing, sewing through the fold (by hand or machine), and double-fan adhesive binding. Each technique has its advantages and disadvantages, and its appropriateness is dependent upon the item and its intended use. Primary factors driving the leaf attachment decision are paper quality, inner margin width, presence of an acceptable sewing structure, and whether the leaves are single or folded signatures [27].

Oversewing

Once the mainstay of library binding, oversewing has lost its privileged position in current practice but continues to be a useful binding option, especially for paper stock that resists glue penetration. In oversewing, 1/8 inch of the inner margin is milled, holes are punched, and threaded needles are passed through the textblock; then threads are crosswoven horizontally up the spine. The fundamental arguments against the technique are that it reduces openability, uses up more inner margin than other methods, increases chances for damage from photocopying due to tight construction, and increases chances that weakened paper will tend to break where stitched [28]. More generally useful alternatives are now thought to be sewing through the fold, double-fan adhesive binding, and recasing (i.e., reusing the original page attachment structure in a rebuilt case).

Sewing Through the Fold

Sewing through the fold is used primarily on serials in which leaves are gathered in signatures—sheets folded vertically down their centers and joined by thread or staples. Familiar journals such as *Lancet, Scientific American*, and *BMJ* are examples of signature construction. Whether done by hand or machine, sewing through the fold allows for optimal openability and requires no sacrifice of inner margins, since no milling is done. However, a major disadvantage may be the cost passed on to the library for the skill that is required by bindery personnel for this technique.

Double-fan Adhesive Binding

This is the most readily applied method of leaf attachment and one that has gained favored status in current practice. The process entails milling a small amount of spine to remove the original glued binding and to align the leaves, and then notching the edge to provide more surface area for glue adhesion. The volume is clamped in a machine and the leaves are fanned in one direction. A thin layer of polyvinyl acetate (PVA) adhesive is applied to the page edges, and fanning is then done in the reverse direction with more glue applied. A thin, stretchy cloth lining is then placed over the glued spine and partly overlapped onto the endsheets. The adhesive is slow drying and stays flexible, unlike the animal-based glues used by publishers for softcover books and journal issues. Because many scientific journals are produced on glossy, clay-coated paper, which does not allow the adhesive to penetrate completely, volumes that get high use may have a greater tendency to lose pages than oversewn volumes.

Quality Control

No matter what leaf attachment methods are used, a library should continuously monitor the condition of bound volumes and communicate with its binder if loose pages or broken bindings are common. Many problems can be resolved by altering the leaf attachment method or by binding fewer issues in a single volume. Librarians are well advised to stay current with emerging issues in binding technology through professional journals such as the *New Library Scene* (available as a free subscription through many commercial binders) and by regular meetings with binder representatives. To help fully understand the techniques, there is no substitute for visiting a bindery in operation. Some controversial issues that librarians need to be aware of since they may be viewed differently by different binders are the comparative benefits of trimming versus no-trim policies, rounding and backing versus flat-backed spines, and flush bottom versus recessed case construction.

Binding Contracts

One way to establish the responsibilities of both the library and the binder is through a formal contract. Even if institutional authorities do not require a formal, written agreement, it is a good way to get products and services for a set price, as well as convey the library's needs and expectations. The basic contract elements for binding services are the anticipated number of volumes to be bound, the price-per-volume for each type of binding or repair, the charges for extra services, and the turnaround time [29]. The technical specifications as established should explicitly address collation standards, page repairs, permissible methods of leaf attachment, material standards for cover construction, trimming, rounding and backing, recasing, spine lettering, and the use of special nonstandard treatments. The binder should demonstrate its ability to meet the terms of the contract by supplying names of current clients, a sample of its work, and a written warranty of compliance to LBI Standards. LBI offers a Pre-Contract Book Examination Service that, for a small fee, allows a library to submit volumes to the Dudley A. Weiss Book Testing Laboratory at the Rochester Institute of Technology for examination and an impartial evaluation [30].

Contract terms should cover insurance, pickup and delivery schedules, binding slips, responsibility for correcting errors, automated services, and invoice terms [31-32]. Ideally, a librarian familiar with the binding process, rather than a purchasing agent, should write the contract, and then educate the purchasing agent to the importance of quality products and services as opposed to rewarding the contract to the lowest bidder. The advice of Gordon and Jacobsen in drafting commercial binding agreements is sound: sample existing models from other institutions, talk to knowledgeable librarians and binders, use the LBI Standards, attend workshops, read articles, and use common sense [33].

Automation and Binding

Automation of bindery-related library processes comes in various forms and levels of sophistication, as it does for other serials control functions. Libraries have developed in-house systems, used binder-developed systems, or have implemented binding components in serials control systems from subscription agencies, bibliographic utilities, and integrated library systems (ILS) vendors [34-38]. Generally, automated binding systems should

- Identify and print lists of items ready to be considered for binding.
- Store title-specific nonvariable binding data.
- Print binding slips.
- Print binding shipment packing lists.
- Update the location and status of items during the binding process.
- Retain records of bound volumes.
- Track fiscal expenditures related to binding.
- Generate reports on binding activities.

It is fair to say, however, that all existing binding systems have limitations, in that all lack some fundamental element that would complete the coordinated cycle of information flow between library and bindery. In attempts to gain efficiency with dwindling resources, as Jacobsen states, "some librarians are willing to investigate any technological solution that is offered to them by aggressive salesmen, without really evaluating the effects that such technology will have on their organizations" [39]. As harsh as this may sound, technology-driven systems for binding that easily entice librarians are no exception to this phenomenon.

Academic health sciences libraries, with their large serials collections in proportion to the size of their serials staffs, are good candidates for automating bindery-related processes. However, libraries that are required to bid binding services on a regular basis should not invest heavily in proprietary, binder-developed systems, but should instead choose systems that are created in-house or are modules of ILS software, or have broad support in the binding industry. Whatever the choice, libraries should encourage and support the development and use of industry-wide standards.

Probably the most widely used system currently is Advanced Bindery/Library Exchange (ABLE). Developed in 1985 by Mekatronics/Bendor International, Inc., ABLE is recognized as the current industry "standard" in automated binding systems. Aiding processing at both the library and the bindery, it is an IBM-compatible microcomputer-based program that relies on disks to transfer information between the library and the bindery. The advantages for the library are that it eliminates filing and storing preprinted binding slips, allows the library to add, change or delete titles from its database, and requires little training to learn. The system shows binding histories for titles, provides report-generating capabilities, and interfaces library data with binder's data for spine lettering [40].

An important drawback of the system is that it requires libraries to add yet another stand-alone automated system, requiring ongoing maintenance and training. It also puts a greater onus of responsibility on the library for getting the spine stamping and other instructions correct. In addition, the library shares responsibility with the binder for backing up and maintaining the database of binding data specific to the library. Many advantages and efficiencies accrue to the commercial binder when a library begins to supply binding instructions in machine-readable form; in return, libraries should reasonably expect improvements in binding accuracy and turnaround time, if not reduced charges.

Library-developed automated binding systems have proven useful for various steps in binding preparation, including generation of binding slips and shipment lists [41-42]. More popular, however, have been the binding modules of integrated library systems. The movement toward building binding processes into integrated library systems began in the 1980s, but, as late as 1992, most systems did not support a core list of desirable functions for binding [43]. All systems have had partial components at best. A few of them offered streamlined record-keeping, provided automatic notification of volumes ready to be bound, and linked binding status to online public catalogs. As pressures to upgrade and enhance other features of ILS systems grew more intense, binding dropped as a priority on the list of planned enhancements. Consequently, there are many systems that have only partially developed binding components. To develop the ideal system would take the cooperative efforts of binders, librarians, and system designers in establishing standards and undertaking a comprehensive plan of action.

The greatest hope lies in the development of industry-wide standard protocols to facilitate the exchange of binding-related information. An ALA committee, the Automation Vendor Information and Advisory Committee (AVIAC), with its working committee on Communication of Binding Information, is coordinating efforts with the Serials Industry Systems Advisory Committee (SISAC) and the Book Industry Systems Advisory Committee (BISAC) to speed automation in binding by developing standard record formats to be used between systems [44]. The basic elements for the generic interface are the X12 standards for electronic data interchange (EDI) that will allow library automated binding systems to communicate with binders' automated systems. After defining the data elements for communication, the proposal will be submitted to the National Information Standards Organization (NISO). By bringing together the major stakeholders to develop standard formats for binding information, and at the same time building upon both the X12 and ANSI Z39.2-1992 (Information Interchange) standards, it is hoped that the time period for their creation and acceptance will be shortened [45].

Alternatives to Permanent Binding

Medical libraries typically bind the majority of journals they receive, with the exception of those titles that are retained for a limited period of time, including titles for which a microform subscription is also maintained and titles that are of ephemeral interest and significance. Low-use titles may be bound in nonstandard bindings that most binders offer as part of their special services.

In major medical research collections of considerable age, it is important that library personnel be able to identify deteriorated material that should not be given standard library binding, both for the good of the items and in the interest of conserving funds for binding other items. In libraries housing such collections, it is increasingly expected that library staff responsible for binding be able to properly judge the condition of materials, and know that normal library binding is inappropriate for brittle material. Alternative approaches such as replacement volumes, phase boxing or other protective enclosures, reformatting to acid-free paper, relying on microfilm or a digitized format, or simple withdrawal are options to be weighed against the intrinsic value, predicted future use, and estimated value of the volumes as part of the entire collection. Overall, a conservative approach to preservation of deteriorated materials is often the most prudent one. In the words of a preservation librarian, "It is much better to do nothing to a volume than to damage it through improper binding or rebinding techniques and materials" [46].

Recasing, i.e., attaching an existing binding to new boards, can be done for sewn-signature volumes when the sewing and textblock is intact, even though the paper may be embrittled. The binder cleans the old glue away, attaches new endsheets, and constructs a new case. This method is recommended when the volume's condition permits, since it requires no milling of margins and preserves openability. But, it can be a labor-intensive procedure for the binder that may cost the library more to have done.

For low-use titles, long-term retention of unbound issues is an alternative, but one that must be cautiously evaluated, since, "in most cases, it is not possible to reduce the number of items needing binding without creating an organizational crisis of loose periodical parts vulnerable to theft and loss" [47]. The University of Texas Health Center Library at Tyler experienced such a crisis when it tried to maintain five years of unbound issues while converting to microfilm for space reasons. After just two years, it discovered that high frequency titles like *Lancet* and *JAMA* suffered loss of issues and loss of ordered control, and binding was resumed [48]. Alternative in-house binding methods such as comb or spiral binding, pin or tack binding, pambinding, thermal machine binding, and the VeloBind process may be used, but mixed results at large academic libraries suggest that most health sciences libraries probably would not benefit from using these techniques [49].

In-House Repairs

Automation enables libraries to reduce the staff time expended in bindery preparation, thus freeing personnel to do, among other tasks, in-house repairs such as tipping in loose pages, reinforcing broken hinges, and mending torn pages—costly services when performed by the binder. Besides the direct cost savings, the library may be more selective in the materials and methods used for repairs and develop a comprehensive preservation program that is better for collection maintenance. For instance, rather than accept the use of pressure-sensitive tape in repairs by binders, the library may choose to mend tears with Japanese paper and carefully selected glues. Heavily used journals will be returned to the shelves sooner and be more accessible than if they were sent to the bindery for such repairs. Also, by training a staff member to do simple repairs, the library will guard against those creative but damaging quick fixes done by the preservationally unenlightened members of the staff [50]. Adequate space, materials, trained personnel, and administrative support must be provided for in-house repair units in order for them to be successful. Several excellent introductions to library repair techniques are available [51-54].

Holdings and Locations Statements

Although individual serials generally follow set publication patterns, as a format serials are notorious for the myriad variations by which their items may be identified. Holdings statements describe the range of items or the specific items that the library has acquired, inventoried, and retains in its collection. The creation and maintenance of serials holdings information can be a daunting task for librarians who seek to record and then communicate this information. Borrowing words from Grosch, "the purpose of any serial holding statement is to convey useful information to those who either operate, depend upon, or use the data to verify or locate a specific serial issue reference" [55]. To do so, holdings appear in alphabetic journal holdings lists, as a part of the bibliographic records in online catalogs, as a component in automated serials control systems, and on "holdings cards" in libraries that still maintain card catalogs and serials shelflists.

The typical elements that comprise holdings statements are journal volume and issue enumeration and chronological designations. The level of specificity and complexity of holdings statements depends on the intended use and on system parameters, whether manual or automated. Holdings formats may take various forms, but generally fall into two basic categories: summary and detailed holdings. Some examples of holdings statements in Table 4-3 illustrate the common elements and possible variations in format that exist.

Accurate holdings statements depend upon accurate linkages to the full bibliographic records. Title changes, cessations, and withdrawals necessitate actions for updating holdings in serials records. Since the current standard for successive entry cataloging requires individual catalog records for each title, the current practice for holdings data is to attach only the items that fall within the title's bibliographic scope. As a result, a single serial publication may be reflected by several linked records, with each record having its own holdings.

Guaranteeing that accurate title connections are provided through notes and linking entries and that each record displays only those items covered chronologically in the title description is demanding work requiring close coordination between cataloging and serials records staff. Integrating procedures for holdings updating into routine serials acquisitions work flow also ensures that holdings records correctly reflect new subscriptions, lost or missing journal issues, added backfiles, changes in retention policy, or withdrawn volumes. Attention to detail and good communications with other library units are vital to proper holdings reporting. Accuracy and consistency are not the hobgoblins of this activity; they are the heart of the matter.

Machine-readable serials holdings that are integrated into online public access catalogs offer the best opportunity for maintaining accurate holdings, since many more eyes view, interpret, and provide feedback to the serials staff. Retrospective serials holdings may be created by inventorying physical items piece-by-piece and then keying the data into the system, or by the more common practice of converting and loading an earlier machine-readable holdings database, such as a union list, by magnetic tape.

Table 4-3: Examples of Summary Holdings Statements

UCI Biomed W1 JA163 B174-270:1-8(1960-93); Current Issues on Display
Shelves.
UCI MedCtr W1 JA163 B174-268(1960-92)U269N1-12(1993); Current Issues
on Display Shelves.

BSU PERIOD STACKS v.199-239(1967-1978)v.267(1992)-
BSU PER CALL#:R15.A48
BOUND v.183- (1963-
MICROFILM v.173#9-182 (1960-62)

TSU PER
CURRENT ISSUES DISPLAYED
V.248 (1982)-V.266 NO.16(1991);V.267(1992)- BOUND
V.266 NO.17-24(1991)INCOMPLETE & UNBOUND

UMBC SERIAL STACKS
v.142(1950)-v.150(1950);v.172-173(1960);
v.183(1963)-v.217(1971);v.219(1972)-v.225(1973)
v.227(1974)-v.234(1975); v.238(1977)-

MUSC Copy 1:
Hold: SHELVED AS: JOURNAL OF THE AMERICAN MEDICAL ASSOCIATION.
HOLD: 1960-1993 : 173N9-17/174-269/270N1-19/

Standards

To aid in communicating holdings information, national standards have
been established. The current national standard for holdings statements
under review, the American National Standard, Holdings Statements for
Bibliographic Items, Z39.71, has developed through the consolidation of its
predecessors:

- Serial Holdings Statements at the Summary Level, Z39.42-1980.

- Serial Holdings Statements at the Detailed Level.

- Serial Holdings Statements, Z39.44-1986.

- Holdings Statements for Non-Serial Holdings, Z39.57-1989.

ANSI sets the standards, and the USMARC Format for Holdings and
Locations provides format specifications for implementation. Based on the
development of Serial Holdings Statements, ANSI Z39.44-1986, the US-

MARC format provides the means for standard communication of holdings data. For a review of holding statements implementations and insight into future developments, *The USMARC Format for Holdings and Locations: Development, Implementation and Use,* edited by Barry B. Baker, is recommended [56]. Adherence to these evolving national standards substantially aids in the sharing of holdings data for cooperative products such as union lists and Internet-accessible catalogs.

New Directions

Some of the most exciting developments in holdings recording and transmission are going on in ways that are invisible to most library users. Summary holdings generated automatically from local check-in records are being transmitted to state, regional, and national levels with increasing transparency. Holdings data are also being linked behind the scene to article level records in indexing and abstracting databases. For instance, locally mounted MEDLINE databases now may indicate in each citation whether a journal source is in the local library collection. Typically this link is done at the title level, but future developments may permit more precise matching between article citations and the library's detailed holdings information. The potential for the Serial Item and Contribution Identifier (SICI) to act as a universal connector is being explored by SISAC.

Union Listing

Union listing is the product of cooperative agreements to coordinate and pool serials bibliographic and holdings data from multiple institutions into one source for the purposes of resource sharing, cooperative collection development, preservation, and interlibrary loan. Union lists continue to be valuable tools, especially as libraries increasingly explore cooperative access to low-use titles. According to Hepfer "significant factors in the boom in union listing include the availability of bibliographic records from the CONSER database, the continued improvement of telecommunications technology, the development and widespread adoption of the ANSI Standard for Serial Holdings Statements at the Summary Level, and the trend toward resource sharing among libraries" [57]. Health science libraries of all kinds and sizes, with their strong nationwide network organized through the National Library of Medicine, have a rich history of cooperative union listing agreements. Such arrangements occur on local, state, regional, and national levels with their resulting compilations appearing in paper, COM (computer output microform), magnetic tape, CD-ROM, and online data files.

Union listing is synonymous with compromise, and major concerns beset libraries when combining and sharing data. Issues that must be addressed include

- Overall goals and purposes.

- Levels of commitment and participation.

- Centralized or decentralized administration.

- Allocation of costs.

- Scope of inclusion by subject or format.

- Bibliographic authority for title entry.

- Inclusion of multiple versions of titles.

- Holdings statement formats.

- Quality control and error correction.

- Updating schedule and frequency.

- Method of compilation (manual or automated).

- Generation and forms of products.

Health sciences libraries are active participants in a wide range of consortial union listing groups that represent everything from subject-focused groups that are exclusively biomedical in nature, to multitype library groups that cross subject and geographic boundaries. To manage the data and generate the output, libraries employ the services of commercial firms or other libraries, utilize capabilities in their networked serials control systems, or design and create their own products with microcomputer programs.

SERHOLD

The literature on union listing in medical libraries seems to provide as many different consortial configurations and kinds of lists as there are titles in them [58-61]. However, the premier cooperative program among health sciences libraries is SERHOLD, a machine-readable serials holdings database of 40,000 serials titles and about 1,300,000 holdings statements, contributed by approximately 3,150 U.S. and selected Canadian biomedical libraries [62]. SERHOLD is used today to generate many, if not most U.S.

regional biomedical union lists. The database was created in 1981 by NLM with the cooperation of the Regional Medical Libraries, and other individual biomedical libraries. At that time, medical libraries already had an interlibrary loan network, but as a result of SERHOLD, NLM was able to implement the DOCLINE system for automatic routing of ILL requests.

According to Bloss, "the availability of high quality serial bibliographic records provides the first component in any vision of union list activities" [63]. This underlying requirement was amply met in the SERHOLD system, since NLM's SERLINE records, each with its own unique title control number and automatically generated cross-references, became the bibliographic authority for SERHOLD. NLM creates and maintains all bibliographic data, stores and processes the machine-readable holdings data from the participants, and produces the machine-readable data used for products from the bibliographic and holdings data. The coordinators at designated regional libraries collect and transfer this data, while individual libraries identify and update their holdings by reporting data [64].

SERHOLD's scope is defined by NLM as "currently published or ceased journals in the fields of biomedicine, health care delivery, natural sciences, life sciences and related topics or peripheral subjects such as botany, agriculture, general education, mathematics, linguistics, statistics and administration and management journals which assist in health care delivery" [65]. In recent years, NLM has allowed libraries to report holdings for journals that are not in NLM's collection. As a result, more journals in subject areas such as computer and library science, chemistry, business, veterinary science, and agriculture have been added.

Similar to other union lists, SERHOLD maintains holdings at the volume level not the issue level, and incomplete volumes are not reported. Currently the ANSI Z39.42-1986 Serial Holdings Statements standard with some revision provides a common format for direct transmission of holdings data to SERHOLD. However, libraries, even within the same region and sometimes within a library for different titles, are permitted to report at various levels. As of April 1995, 91% of the holdings were entered at summary level 3, the recommended level for DOCLINE routing [66]. Level 3 supplies the library symbol, date of report, acquisition status code, and volume and year in standard format. Level X denotes a nonstandard format for the same elements and accounted at that time for 9% of the database [67]. For the future, since most document requests can be routed accurately based on summary holdings data, NLM has no plans to use detailed level 4 holdings in SERHOLD. In addition to the SERHOLD format, NLM also accepts holdings data in the OCLC MARC format and USMARC format. Table 4-4 illustrates standard SERHOLD holdings formats.

In October 1993, NLM introduced an online updating system to be used by contributing libraries for viewing, adding, updating, and deleting SERHOLD records. To encourage accurate and timely holdings submissions

Table 4-4: Examples of SERHOLD Holdings Statements

Level 2:
02JHU (920514 2R)
02JHU (920524 2)

Level 3:
[Holdings Permanently Retained]
02JHU (920504 3R)1-.1976-
02JHU (920505 3)1-6,88.1950-1955,1957
02JHU (920504 3).1984-

[Holdings Retained for a Limited Period]
02JHU (92050463 , LAST 3 YEARS)
02JHU (92050463 , CURRENT YEAR ONLY)

Level X:
02JHU (920504 X)V.1-
02JHU (920504 X)1,1971-2
02JHU (920505 X)4-5N3;6N2-8(1974-1978
02JHU (920504 X)Library retains last two years

(Adapted from: Format for Direct Transmission of Holdings Data to the National Library of Medicine's SERHOLD Database. National Library of Medicine, rev. 9/22/92, p.12-3.)

---

from participating libraries, most regional union list coordinators and SERHOLD reporting agencies have stipulated that any library that fails to update its SERHOLD holdings in two consecutive years will be deleted from the database and DOCLINE participation. Here again is evidence of the impact of serials work on other library functions and services.

Network Cooperation: NLM and OCLC

The large bibliographic utilities, such as OCLC, Research Libraries Information Network (RLIN), and the Washington Library Network (WLN), were also instrumental in the development of union listing. OCLC, in particular, has developed an extensive union listing component and affords health sciences libraries an alternative means for SERHOLD updating. About a dozen health sciences groups report to SERHOLD through OCLC union listing. The groups range from a few libraries in central New York to over 350 libraries in the Greater Midwest Region of the National Network of Libraries of Medicine.

The foundation of current OCLC/NLM SERHOLD links dates to 1986 when a group of Michigan health sciences libraries created the Michigan Statewide Health Sciences Union List of Serials (MISHULS) with OCLC's union listing system [68]. Standard OCLC MARC union list data was programmed by NLM to convert to SERHOLD format; this capability was offered to other libraries with the 1987 update. This experience is an example of a biomedical group operating as a subset of a state multitype union listing consortium. Such a model offers the advantages of decentralized input, access to a wider range of resources for ILL, and holdings that are keyed only once. Building upon the work of this pioneering group, Alabama health sciences libraries furthered the OCLC-SERHOLD connection by developing refinements in selection of bibliographic records, assignment of OCLC holdings symbols, tape processing between OCLC and NLM, sequencing of union listing products, and in the utilization of exception reports from NLM tape loads. These were areas identified as being in need of further collaboration among individual participants, OCLC, and NLM [69-70].

Tapeloading of serials union listing data from OCLC to SERHOLD has continued to progress. However, an area that remains problematic is tapeloading local system holdings data into the OCLC union listing system, since OCLC has not yet developed batch processing through tapes for record maintenance. Tapeloading into OCLC can only be done to create records, not to modify or delete records; changes to existing records must be made online. OCLC is presently working on this enhancement as part of its implementation of the USMARC holdings format in its PRISM software. OCLC has loaded a few files, one being that from the Greater Midwest Region of the National Network of Libraries of Medicine [71]. As networked gateways connect interlibrary loan systems and other databases in the future, many of the current administrative challenges to union listing projects should be alleviated.

Future of Union Listing

As the purposes, forms, participants, and nature of union lists evolve within libraries, some seers predict the eventual passing of these noble collective undertakings. Others see their basic concepts evolving into new ways of organizing the vast amount of holdings data on the Internet, as global networks give union catalogs new meaning [72]. Automated serials control modules of ILS systems are beginning to reflect some of these new needs by providing for consortial use of a single system [73]. Printed union lists may indeed go the way of the dinosaurs, but the same underlying strategies will evolve into more accessible, multilibrary networked holdings databases.

Networked automated union lists may well provide better pathways for cooperative collection development, resource sharing, and preservation projects. Holdings data linked across networks can make possible future routing systems for document delivery of electronic full text documents, provided that the level of reporting moves from title-level to article-level holdings. The 1980s may be said to have been the decade of union listing, but the 90s and beyond may be the era when this activity blossoms into new forms.

Special Serials Services

Errata and Retractions

As respected journals increasingly establish consistent policies on publishing errata and retractions, librarians need to develop policies and procedures for identifying them, incorporating them into local databases, and recording them in the journal issues themselves. Errata and retractions arise from distinctly different conditions and are defined differently. An erratum is a statement of change or emendation, sometimes called a correction or corrigendum, that is published by a publisher, editor, or author in reference to a previously published article, and results from substantive typographical or other inadvertent errors identified after the article is printed. A retraction is a notice of an article that has been retracted, disavowed, or withdrawn by the authors, academic or institutional sponsor, editor, or publisher, because of pervasive error or unsubstantiated or irreproducible data [74]. Articles are retracted because of faulty conclusions due to honest errors in logic, miscomputations, and contaminated data, or due to scientific misconduct such as falsified or fabricated data or plagiarism.

Readers assume published data are accurate unless informed otherwise. Errors in the administration and dosages of therapeutic drugs or predicted surgical outcomes based on incorrect data may lead to treatments that have lethal consequences. Although the percentage of errors in publication is small in relation to the high number of published studies in biomedicine, the potential of spreading misinformation is substanatially magnified through subsequent citations and incorporation in textbooks and teaching [75].

Whether the errors are unintentional or not, the library's policy to assist users of the literature in identifying such errors is viewed by some librarians as bordering on censorship, while others see it as their responsibility to warn of misinformation. Certainly the ultimate responsibility for assessing the validity and accuracy of the information lies with the user of the health sciences literature. Librarians, however, need to formulate library policy for determining the course of local action related to their collections. The decision to tag original articles within the physical journal issues is best made cooperatively by library administration, collection management librarians, and public services staff. When the choice is to implement a local retraction and errata tagging program, the responsibility may fall with the serials department or be a cooperative effort between reference and serials personnel.

In some libraries, practices and policies on errata and retractions have been formalized in recent years, yet many U.S. medical libraries still do not identify or have policies to handle the invalid articles in their collections [76]. Libraries which may lack an organized program in this area, usually do, however, attach or write in information from separate errata notices mailed by publishers. Some current policies of medical libraries for handling these error notices are summarized in an article by Cooper [77].

It has become increasingly convenient to identify and track such information because of the policies established by NLM. For errata identification, NLM amends each citation in MEDLINE when its associated article has had a citable erratum published. To qualify as a citable erratum, the notice must appear on a numbered page within the journal, and not be issued as a separate piece to be tipped in. The bibliographic reference for the erratum notice is added to the original article citation. Although errata must be citable, NLM does not index errata notices as separate articles unless they are substantive articles or letters.

For retraction identification, NLM tags citations in MEDLINE only when articles have been unequivocally declared by the author, by the author's legal representative, by the sponsoring agency, or by the journal editor to be a retracted article. Like errata notices, the condition that a retraction appears in a citable form must also hold true, in order to be tagged in MEDLINE. Unlike most errata, retraction notices are indexed, and, in addition, carry a Publication Type of "Retraction of Publication." To ensure the linkage to the original publication, the MEDLINE citation for each retracted article is tagged as Publication Type "Retracted Publication." The title information in both citations is also amended with the bibliographic citation to its counterpart.

Many libraries have devised strategies for identifying and marking retracted articles in their collections. Routinely updating a search of MEDLINE for the Publication Type "Retracted Publication" provides citations to articles that can then be tagged in their physical volumes by stamping an alerting notice or by tipping in a citation for the retraction. When planning local policy for errata and retractions, it is important to fully understand NLM's policies for identifying them [78]. The most current information is available from the Chief, Bibliographic Services Division, National Library of Medicine, Bethesda, MD 20894.

Public Service Assistance

A strong case for using serials specialists as intermediaries between the collection and users is made by Pinzelik in a thorough examination of the complexities users encounter in accessing serial literature within collections [79]. There exists an innate relationship between reference and serials work, which has only intensified with the increased accessibility of electronically distributed abstracting and indexing databases and table of contents services. For this reason, users benefit when reference and serials staff work in tandem.

Interpreting questions not only at the reference desk but at any library service point can often benefit from the unique familiarity that serials specialists develop with the serials collection. Participation of serials staff in public assistance can also help to relieve some of the pressure on reference staff caused by their expanding instructional responsibilities. Placing serials staff at service points sensitizes them to real user problems and needs, and becomes a strategy for enhancing serials records and services from the users' perspective. Whether or not serials staff members are formally integrated into public service activities, ongoing two-way communication between public service staff and serials staff is essential.

Special Services

The trend in libraries is toward customizing services to satisfy the needs of individuals or specific user groups. In the area of serials acquisition, hospital libraries have traditionally offered services to their users in entering and maintaining journal subscriptions for departmental or personal use. Depending on the expertise of the serials staff and the level of administrative support, in-house book repair services, centralized binding for departmental collections, and searches for replacement issues can be valuable services to individual users, as well as important public relations opportunities. With the wealth of information residing within library automated systems, librarians can also produce reports on their collections that can aid individuals in accreditation procedures, grant funding, research, teaching, and administration.

Serials-related services can include tailored current awareness alerts such as prepublication table of contents distribution coupled with document delivery services. Libraries may also choose to transmit to individuals or departments electronic notices of the day's journal receipts and descriptions of newly acquired serials titles or titles being considered for acquisition. Many libraries now have the capability to deliver full-text electronic journals to individuals' electronic mail addresses and to guarantee authenticated archival versions for future reference. As the focus moves to defining services for users and away from overseeing processing functions, serials operations will need to reconsider priorities and realign staffing accordingly. Evaluating and reorganizing collections and services to better serve users will result in a revitalization of all serials management activities.

Future of Serials Management

Change is.nothing new to serials work. Librarians who have managed serials have acquired, perhaps by osmosis, a transformational nature that adapts itself well to serials operations in transitional times. However, only the naive think that moving from manual systems for controlling print collections to managing services related to electronic serials on the Internet will be a matter of routine. While still facing familiar serials management dilemmas, tomorrow's serials librarian will be confronted with a broad range of new challenges requiring cooperative approaches and the forging of new partnerships beyond the library's walls.

As users learn to exploit the functionality of electronic journals and electronic periodical databases, serials specialists in health sciences libraries will be called upon to explore remote boundaries of the library universe and to reshape services tailored to radically new needs. Just as the cataloging, check-in, claiming, inventorying, routing, arranging, union listing, binding, and preserving of print serials collections dominated the past century, the creating, transmitting, organizing, displaying, and archiving of electronic journals will consume the next. Links between print and electronic collections, and between source material and custom-designed indexes, will become increasingly sophisticated, with document delivery on-demand a driving force. The integration of all processes related to serials management and use will require new policies and paradigms in the library, its parent institution, and the scholarly community as a whole. Looking at old problems in new ways will be an essential skill, but identifying new problems inherent in proposed solutions will be equally necessary. Whether or not libraries are fully prepared for them, advancing technologies will continue to redesign serials and their management.

References

1. Smith TE. Using a serials control system in a reference setting. Inf Technol Libr 1986 Jun;5(2):135-40.

2. Puccio JA. Serials reference work. Englewood, CO: Libraries Unlimited, 1989.

3. Kinder R, Katz B, eds. Serials and reference services. New York: Haworth Press, 1990.

4. LaCroix EM. Survey on journal arrangement—summary. In: MEDLIB-L [electronic bulletin board]. Start N, system operator. Buffalo (NY): State University of New York;1993 Feb 26.

5. Tuttle M. Introduction to serials management. Greenwich, CT: JAI Press, 1983.

6. Thornton GA. Physical access to periodical literature: the dilemma revisited and a brief look at the future. Ser Rev 1991 Winter;17(4):33-42.

7. Medical Library Association. MLA Exchange Advisory Committee. Request for information to automate the Medical Library Association Serials Exchange. Apr 11,1991:1-10.

8. Geller M. Duplicate exchange list. In: MEDLIB-L [electronic bulletin board]. Start N, system operator. Buffalo (NY): State University of New York; 1994 Sept 29.

9. Cooper ER. Options for the disposal of unwanted donations. Bull Med Libr Assoc 1990 Oct;78(4):388-94.

10. Fisher JS. Smithsonian phases out international exchange service. MLA News 1992 Nov/Dec;(250):8.

11. Cooper ER, op. cit., 393-4.

12. American Council of Learned Societies. Manual for international book and journal donations. Greenberg, J., comp. New York: American Council of Learned Societies, 1993.

13. Ruelle B. International donation of medical journals and books: a how-to manual. Med Ref Serv Q 1992 Summer;11(2):35-43.

14. Jaeger D. Back-volume acquisitions: an historical perspective. Tech Serv Q 1987 Summer;4(4):33-8.

15. Directory of back issue dealers. Holley, B., comp. Decatur,GA: North American Serials Interest Group, 1991.

16. Garno V. USBE: recycling resources. ASIS Bull 1983 Feb;9:18-9.

17. Makinen R. Our binding dilemma. Biomed Libr Bull 1991 Apr;(107):1.

18. National Library of Medicine. Preservation Section. Methods of library binding. Bethesda, MD: National Library of Medicine, 1988:1-3.

19. Byrnes MM. Preservation of the biomedical literature: an overview. Bull Med Libr Assoc 1989 Jul;77(3):269-75.

20. Walker G. Library binding as a conservation measure. Collect Manage 1982 Spring/Summer;4(1/2):55-71.

21. Campbell GR. Toward a new standard for library binding. New Libr Scene 1994 Aug;13(4):5-6.

22. Library Binding Institute. Library Binding Institute standard for library binding. 7th ed. Boston: Library Binding Institute, 1981.

23. Parisi PA, Merrill-Oldham J, eds. Library Binding Institute standard for library binding. 8th ed. Rochester, NY: Library Binding Institute, 1986.

24. Merrill-Oldham J, Parisi P. Guide to the Library Binding Institute standard for library binding. Chicago: American Library Association, 1990.

25. Parisi PA. New directions in library binding—life after Class A: technical considerations: 1986 LBI standard. New Libr Scene 1992 Apr;11(2)10-11,23-4.

26. Morrow CC. The preservation challenge: a guide to conserving library materials. White Plains, NY : Knowledge Industry, 1983.

27. Parisi PA. Methods of affixing leaves: options and implications. New Libr Scene 1994 Feb;13(1):8-11,15.

28. Roberts M. Oversewing and the problem of book preservation in the research library. Coll Res Libr 1967 Jan;28(1):17-24.

29. Weiss DA. A checklist for buying library binding. New Libr Scene 1984 Apr;3(2):16,18.

30. Lazar JH. Bidding library binding. New Libr Scene 1988 Oct;7(5):1,5.

31. McCrady E. Guide to drafting of contracts. Special supplement on library binding. Abbey News 1984 Feb;8(1pt2):13-6.

32. Grauer S. Report on bidding library binding contracts. New Libr Scene 1988 Aug;7(4):11.

33. McAdam T. The Commercial binding agreement: partners in preservation. Ser Libr 1990;17(3/4):153-4.

34. Hoskins MB, Reid MT. Online communication with binders: the Hertzberg connection. Ser Libr 1985 Summer;9(4):83-7.

35. Townsend T. Automated bindery preparation: the Hertzberg connection at Iowa State. Ser Rev 1985 Winter;11(4):51-5.

36. Campbell HH, Boomgaarden WL. The Ohio State University libraries' utilization of General Bookbinding Company's automated binding records system. Ser Rev 1986 Winter;12(4):89-99.

37. Forsman RB. EBSCONET serials control system: a case history and analysis. Ser Rev 1982 Winter;8(4):83-5.

38. Greenberg E. OCLC's serials subsystem: success at CWRU. Ser Rev 1982 Winter;8(4):77-81.

39. Jacobsen B. Computer communications and binderies. New Libr Scene 1986 Apr;5(2):1,12.

40. Parisi P. Advanced bindery/library exchange: ready, willing, and...ABLE. Libr Acquis Pract Theory 1988;12(1):81-6.

41. Marx PC, Marx JN. Automating the production of bindery slips. Technicalities 1985 Mar;5(3):15-6.

42. Kim DU. Computer-assisted binding preparation at a university library. Ser Libr 1984 Winter;9(2):35-43.

43. Boss RW. Technical services functionality in integrated library systems. Libr Tech Rep 1992 Jan/Feb;28(1):1-109.

44. Parisi PA. Binding software interface—a top priority. New Libr Scene 1992 Aug;11(4):1,5-6.

45. Michael JJ. Current work on a binding standard. LITA Newsl 1993 Winter;14(1):18.

46. Walker G. op. cit.

47. Dean J. The binding and preparation of periodicals: alternative structures and procedures. Ser Rev 1980 Jul/Sep;6(3):87-90.

48. Craig T. Re:Binding of periodicals. In: MEDLIB-L [electronic bulletin board]. Start N, system operator. Buffalo (NY): State University of New York;1993 Mar 25.

49. Root TA. Inhouse binding in academic libraries. Ser Rev 1989 Fall;15(3):31-40.

50. Milevski RJ, Nainis L. Implementing a book repair and treatment program. Libr Res Tech Ser 1987 Apr/Jun;31(2):159-76.

51. Kyle H. Library materials preservation manual: practical methods for preserving books, pamphlets, and other printed materials. Bronxville, NY: Nicholas T. Smith, 1983.

52. Milevski RJ. Book repair manual. Springfield, IL: Illinois State Library, 1988.

53. Greenfield J. Books, their care and repair. New York, NY: H.W. Wilson, 1983.

54. Morrow CC. Conservation treatment procedures: a manual of step-by-step procedures for the maintenance and repair of library materials. 2d ed. Littleton, CO: Libraries Unlimited, 1986.

55. Grosch AN. Theory and design of serial holding statements in computer-based serials systems. Ser Libr 1977 Summer;1(4):341-52.

56. Baker BB, ed. The USMARC format for holdings and locations: development, implementation and use. New York: Haworth Press, 1988.

57. Hepfer C. Union listing: a literature review. Ser Rev 1988;14(1/2):99-113.

58. Bell CL. A SERLINE-based union list of serials for basic health sciences libraries: a detailed protocol. Bull Med Libr Assoc 1982 Oct;70(4):380-8.

59. Bell CL. A SERLINE-based union list of serials for basic health sciences libraries: an update experience. Bull Med Libr Assoc 1984 Jan;72(1):26-8.

60. Forsman RB. A vendor-supported experiment in union listing. Ser Libr 1985 Summer;9(4):73-82.

61. Peay WJ, Butter KA, Ellis S. Production of a union list of serials using the PHILSOM serials system. Bull Med Libr Assoc 1984 Jan;72(1):28-29.

62. National Library of Medicine. Factsheet. SERHOLD. Bethesda, MD: National Library of Medicine, April 1995.

63. Bloss ME. And in hindsight...the past ten years of union listing. Ser Libr 1985/86 Fall/Winter;10(1/2):141-8.

64. Willmering WJ, Fishel MR, McCutcheon DE. SERHOLD: evolution of the national biomedical serials holdings database. Ser Rev 1988;14(1/2):7-13.

65. National Library of Medicine. SERHOLD Update Guidelines. Bethesda, MD: National Library of Medicine, 1993.

66. National Library of Medicine. Factsheet, op. cit., 2.

67. National Library of Medicine. Format for direct transmission of holdings data to the National Library of Medicine's SERHOLD database. Bethesda, MD: National Library of Medicine, 1993.

68. Sutton LS, Wolfgram PA. Using the OCLC union listing component for a statewide health sciences union list of serials. Bull Med Libr Assoc 1986 Apr;74(2):104-9.

69. Battistella MS, Rodgers PM. Role of a health library association in the development and coordination of a statewide union list of health science serials. Ser Libr 1986 Oct;11(2):75-81.

70. Battistella MS. The OCLC-SERHOLD connection: an evolution in health sciences union listing. Bull Med Libr Assoc 1991 Oct;79(4):370-6.

71. Gillespie G. Summary:uploading/OCLC union list inquiry. In: SERIALST [electronic bulletin board]. MacLennan B, system operator. Burlington, VT: University of Vermont;1993 Jan 27.

72. Schaffner AC, Landesman B, Martin NP, et al. Perspectives on the future of union listing. Ser Rev 1993 Fall;19(3):71-8,94.

73. Boss RW, op. cit., 48.

74. National Library of Medicine. Factsheet. Errata, retraction, duplicate publication and comment policy. Bethesda, MD: National Library of Medicine, 1995.

75. Pfeifer MP, Snodgrass GL. Medical school libraries' handling of articles that report invalid science. Acad Med 1992 Feb;67(2):109-13.

76. Ibid., 109.

77. Cooper ER. Identifying errata and retractions: simplified approaches for serials management. Ser Rev 1992 Winter;18(4):17-20.

78. Kotzin S, Schuyler PL. NLM's practices for handling errata and retractions. Bull Med Libr Assoc 1989 Oct;77(4):337-42.

79. Pinzelik BP. The Serials maze: providing public service for a large serials collection. J Acad Libr 1982 May;8(2):89-94.

5

Acquisition of Audiovisual and Digital Media

Janis F. Brown and David H. Morse

Health sciences libraries of all types commonly hold at least a selection of audiovisual and digital media in their collections, including such items as CD-ROM database products; videocassettes for patient education; microcomputer software; interactive videodisks for anatomical study; audiocassettes for continuing medical education; a variety of other multimedia educational materials; and electronic newsletters, journals, and data files distributed on the Internet. Although it is unlikely that these materials will seriously challenge the predominance of the printed biomedical literature in the near term, it is clear that the importance of these materials is growing rapidly and that emerging technologies will continue to spawn new media formats and applications at an accelerating rate. Indeed a prominent role for digital publication in the dissemintation of scientific literature is now taken as a given in most discussions of scholarly communication at the threshold of the twenty-first century [1-2].

Procedures for acquiring audiovisual and digital media materials can be based upon procedures and policies for acquisition of other types of library materials, as described in the preceding chapters. Handling of CD-ROM subscription titles, for example, can generally follow procedures similar to those for print subscriptions, and processing of nonserial media orders has much in common with ordering and receiving of print monographs. However, some distinct attributes of these media formats and of their distribution channels do merit specialized policies and procedures. Indeed the heterogeneity of available audiovisual and especially digital media materials as compared to printed books and journals demands a uniquely broad range of technical expertise and collaborative effort in the acquisitions process. Equally important, the intangible and transformable character of digital information forms creates a host of new challenges to traditional item-based acquisitions operations [3].

The most obvious of the factors unique to media acquisitions are

- The necessity, in many settings, of working with a different person or group performing the selection.

- The predominance of direct orders and thus the need to accommodate a variety of publisher/distributor policies.

- The need for procedures to manage the previewing process.

- The increased emphasis on licensing arrangements as opposed to outright purchase, especially for digital media.

- The lack of a standardized system of item identification, such as an ISBN.

- The complexity of the items themselves, involving manuals and other supplementary materials, which must be accounted for in the ordering and receiving process.

- The availability of the same title in a variety of versions for different hardware, requiring special care in the order specification process.

The implications of these characteristic media attributes for the organization and management of acquisitions functions will be the focus of discussion in this chapter.

Organizational Issues

In designing a system for media acquisitions in the library, an important first step is to decide whether the acquisitions process will be fully integrated with other library acquisitions functions, i.e. handled primarily by the same staff who perform book and journal acquisitions, or will instead be more closely tied administratively to other media/microcomputer center operations. Arguments can be made for both approaches, and the ultimate decision will be based upon the library's overall approach to integration of media-based services with other library operations, as well as the staff available in each unit. Hospital libraries may find themselves confronting this issue as a choice between handling media acquisitions through the library or instead leaving the responsibility for these materials to the hospital's in-service training or patient education department.

The integrated acquisitions approach has the advantage of exploiting the expertise of acquisitions staff in such areas as use of standard bibliographic description, automated ordering systems, fiscal accounting, and effective communication with other parts of the technical services operation, most notably the cataloging unit. Integrated fiscal reports can be more easily generated, and in cases of hybrid titles combining print and media, there is no opportunity for confusion about which unit is responsible for which titles.

The media center approach, on the other hand, offers offsetting advantages. Because only a few of the important biomedical media publishers and distributors are also involved in book and journal distribution, regular acquisitions staff are unlikely to be as familiar with these sources as media center personnel, who typically develop working relationships with these sources as they perform other responsibilities, such as media selection and faculty consultation. The media selection process frequently involves direct contact with the publisher to discuss issues of content and intended audience as well as to negotiate pricing and licensing issues; this can cause confusion with the media publisher if another office assumes responsibility for the order when it is actually entered.

Additionally, acquiring media items, especially computer software, is greatly aided by technical expertise, current knowledge of the facilities environment, and convenient access to the equipment required to use the materials — all of which are more likely to be at the disposal of media center staff. Finally, some media center operations may be more motivated to handle rush orders and other special processing requests than large acquisitions departments, for whom media orders constitute only a small percentage of the overall workload. (On this point, however, it is worth noting that media staff may be in such demand for public services functions that they may find it difficult to make time for the less-pressing demands of media acquisitions work.)

Regardless of whether media purchases are 1) "mainstreamed" with other formats in the regular library acquisitions process, 2) handled entirely by media/microcomputer center staff, or 3) some combination of the above, the important point is that the division of responsibilities be clearly understood by all of the involved parties and that care be taken to ensure that adequate staff time is allocated to the often time-intensive processes involved in media ordering and receiving. Confusion about responsibilities and jurisdiction can be especially troublesome for recently introduced formats. CD-ROM subscriptions were the major such culprits in the late 1980s, though most libraries now process these titles on a routine basis.

Network-distributed electronic journals and books are posing a similar array of organizational challenges in the 1990s.

Two areas of media acquisitions that are frequently kept separate from the normal acquisitions procedures and handled by administrative, automation, or public services personnel are ordering of general purpose software for library staff use and acquisition of computer files for local mounting, such as MEDLINE or other databases distributed on tape. This approach reflects the fact that these materials are frequently budgeted outside of the normal library materials budget, that they require special negotiation in the area of licensing and multiple-copy discount arrangements, and, in the case of tapes, that they require technical expertise in specifying formats and in verifying their accuracy and completeness upon receipt. Acquisitions staff, however, need at least to be sufficiently aware of these materials to recognize them and to route them correctly. Additionally, arguments have been advanced for acquisitions departments to develop a much fuller range of expertise in handling all digital formats, including computer tapes, if they are to retain their significance in the overall library mission [4].

Once the broad outlines of the organizational structure have been determined, specific functions in the acquisitions process need to be designated and assigned to appropriate staff. Responsibility for the areas listed below should be considered.

- Determining compatibility with existing equipment and ensuring that required versions are fully specified.

- Preorder checking of bibliographic information and searching of library files for items already owned or on order.

- Investigating and negotiating site licensing or identifying other special pricing arrangements.

- Transmitting orders to publishers or distributors.

- Receiving the items and approving invoices.

- Overseeing the preview process (arranging for reviewers to evaluate the items, ensuring that the items are returned in the allotted time).

- Serving as contact person for the vendor to discuss evaluation of the media items.

- Checking the completeness and operability of the items upon arrival.

- Making decisions regarding item packaging, labeling, local mounting, and handling of manuals and other supplementary materials.

- Ensuring that new acquisitions are entered into the appropriate library holdings databases, including serials control systems and catalogs.

In most cases, the responsibility for any given function is placed either on the media selector or on the acquisitions staff, though some functions such as confirming the completeness and operability of the item may also involve cataloging staff. Even with a centralized acquisitions operation, the acquisition process may use media center personnel to assist in determining some of the information needed and in verifying that the correct items have been received before they are passed on to cataloging. The most important consideration is that the responsibilities be unambiguously defined and delegated.

However, consideration should also be given to optimizing the overall acquisitions flow and the efficient processing of the item once it arrives in the library. If different departments are assigned responsibility for different steps in the acquisition process, the process should be designed so that transfers of responsibility from one department to another are kept to a minimum and that record-keeping systems provide adequate tracking of the item throughout the process. Prompt and reliable communication among all of the people involved, including the selector, is the single most critical element in managing the media acquisitions process. The acquisition of free Internet-distributed documents and data files is especially prone to communication gaps, since these files can be downloaded—or simply connected to through a gopher or World Wide Web server—by staff members who are otherwise not involved in acquisitions processes.

Biomedical Media Producers

Before addressing specific operational issues in the acquisitions process, it may be useful to review briefly the various types of organizations involved in the production and distribution of biomedical media. Sources of biomedical media include the largest corporate giants, like Microsoft and McGraw-Hill, as well as the smallest one-person operations — and everything in between. An understanding of the major types of biomedical media publishers is important in designing effective procedures for communicating with these varied organizations and individuals.

General Commercial Publishers

Many of the large commercial publishers of printed biomedical materials, such as Williams & Wilkins, Lippincott, Mosby, and Scientific American, also produce and distribute media items. These are usually the only types of media materials that find their way into the stock of biomedical book vendors and can be ordered in that manner. These materials may be included in the same catalog with the publisher's book and journal publications.

Specialized Commercial Media Publishers

In addition, there are many commercial publishers or distributors that deal only in media items, some of these producing a variety of formats and some limited to only one media format. These include companies like SilverPlatter, Teaching Films, and Audio Digest. Many companies specialize in producing only a single product. For example, DxR Development Group publishes only its clinical case simulation software, *Diagnostic Reasoning*. Information about these companies and their products is generally more difficult to obtain than similar information about the general scientific and technical publishers. These companies can also be expected to be more idiosyncratic in their order fulfillment and pricing policies. Catalogs and product announcements may need to be requested on a regular basis.

Educational Consortia

National and regional consortia and other membership organizations are also sources of media items. Two of the major media consortia are

Health Sciences Consortium
201 Silver Cedar Court
Chapel Hill, NC 27514-1517

Fuld Institute for Technology in Nursing Education
5 Depot Street
Athens, OH 45701

Membership in these organizations provides the library with catalogs of available materials, as well as discounted prices. Special acquisitions procedures may be needed for these materials to ensure that member discounts are correctly applied.

General-Purpose Software Producers

The popular software from producers such as Microsoft, Borland, and Lotus is characterized by its availability through a wide variety of channels, including direct order, mail-order wholesalers, and retail outlets. These producers also commonly provide educational discounts and negotiate institution-wide site licensing agreements with universities and other organizations. Since many of these same products may be ordered by administrative or automation staff for office use, it may be desirable to involve these individuals in their acquisition for the library collection, thereby avoiding unnecessary duplication of effort in comparison shopping and licensing negotiation.

Noncommercial Software

Health sciences faculty, their schools, and universities are also sources of media items, especially computer software. Most typically, a faculty member affiliated with the institution develops a program for use by students and agrees to make it available in the library. The greatest difficulty in handling such items is simply in identifying what they are, since faculty members are generally unconcerned about using consistent titles and version numbers on the labeling and screen displays of these home-grown products.

For faculty-produced software made available to other institutions, contacting the media center at the faculty member's institution may provide the fastest lead to the ordering information. In some cases, faculty-developed software is officially distributed through a departmental office within the school. Here the primary challenge is to get from the selector a complete address, identifying the department or individual to whom the order should be sent. In other cases, home-grown products evolve into commerical enterprises, in which case the products should be ordered in the same way as other commercially produced media.

Pharmaceutical Companies

Pharmaceutical companies are another source of media materials. Through standard acquisitions channels, CIBA-Geigy has long offered the popular slides from the Frank Netter atlases, as well as other slide collections. In addition, some pharmaceutical companies provide computer-based learning materials free of charge to schools and hospitals, usually through direct contact with the media or computer center. Information about available materials can be obtained through the company's professional services department, or its liaisons to medical faculty. These opportunites are becoming less common and not available to all health sciences libraries, but have in the past provided useful educational materials.

Professional Societies and other Organizations

As a component of their publishing services, many professional societies and organizations (e.g., the National League for Nursing, the Radiological Society of North America, the American Society of Clinical Pathologists) sell educational media materials. Their marketing efforts are most likely to be aimed towards members, so requests for purchases may often originate from health professionals and faculty. With sufficient information about the society, the ordering process is straightforward, although prepayment is frequently required.

Network-distributed Software and Data Files

Libraries can also obtain software or other digital data by downloading from Internet FTP sites and electronic bulletin boards or by establishing telnet, gopher, or World Wide Web connections to remote sites. Many of these products are free of charge; others may require one-time or ongoing site licensing payments. As more for-profit companies become connected to the Internet, it seems probable that an increasing percentage of network-distributed sources will require negotiation of payment and licensing terms. As a practical matter, the actual capture or linking of these files may require expertise in network navigation and file transfer on the part of acquisitions staff.

Acquisition Processes

Communication with Selectors and Order Specification

Because media materials are used for a variety of purposes within the library (e.g., as reference information, as educational materials, as office productivity tools), requests for these various types of resources may originate from various departments of the library, most often the reference and media sections, which may control budgeted funds for certain types of material [5]. In some libraries, individuals from departments outside the library may also be authorized to inititate requests for media items. For example, hospital patient education or continuing education departments may serve as the selection agencies for materials that are ordered and maintained by the library.

Since familiarity with different media formats is likely to vary among the different selectors, the acquisitions department needs sufficient expertise to elicit all of the necessary information from the requestor. Complete information concerning media orders is especially important, because the lack of a standard identifier for media materials, such as the ISBN, means that incomplete order specification can easily lead to shipment of the wrong item. In addition to the standard order entry elements, such as title, publisher, date of publication, and estimated price, the media acquisitions request as submitted by the selector should include

- Format of media (e.g., ½" VHS videocassette, 16mm film, microcomputer disk, CD-ROM).

- Whether or not a preview copy is required and who will do the previewing.

- Full address of the producer or distributor, if available.

- Notes on any special publisher/distributor policies already ascertained or negotiated by the selector.

- Notes on special processing requirements (e.g., software to be loaded on network server, faculty member to be notified when item is ready, special library packaging or labeling requirements if known).

In addition, for computer software the selector should also specify

- Computer environment (e.g., DOS, Windows, Macintosh).

- Version number (either a specific number or an indication to purchase the most recent version available).

- Whether or not a network version is needed. (Purchase of a license to use on twenty networked stations is usually different from purchasing twenty individual copies.)

- Number of copies or number of authorized network users. (The requestor should determine if licensing is based upon the number of simultaneous users, the number of computer stations available, or some other criteria.)

A preorder work form specifically for media formats, including the parameters indicated above, may assist in obtaining full information from selectors at the time the request is made. Alternatively, or in addition to the order form, the library may choose to have all media requests routed through the media center to verify that the information is complete and that the materials requested are compatible with current or anticipated library equipment.

Preorder Searching and Verification

In addition to the usual preorder check of library files to ensure that the selected item is not already owned or on order, some preorder research is frequently required to verify or complete the item identification provided by the selector. An especially critical item is the publisher address, since many biomedical media titles are not stocked by the familiar vendors and must be ordered directly from producers or distributors. Unfortunately, bibliographic verification of media materials is often a much more challenging task than it normally is for printed materials, since comprehensive bibliographies and directories are not available for audiovisual and computer software. Also, member-contributed records for media items in the bibliographic utilities such as OCLC and RLIN can be unreliable, and Library of Congress or National Library of Medicine AVLINE records are frequently slow to appear or unavailable.

For these reasons, the library needs to maintain bibliographic resources of its own for media materials, either in the acquisitions department, in the library reference collection, or in the media center. These sources typically include commercially published directories of media titles, individual producer and distributor catalogs, media listings compiled by vendors (Faxon, EBSCO, Majors, and others) and listings of media holdings compiled by other libraries. Lists of suggested verification sources for the various media formats have been compiled by Hayes and Mircheff [6-7]. Some recommended sources are listed in Table 5-1.

If there is any question about the completeness and accuracy of the order information in hand after available reference sources and catalogs have been checked, it is advantageous to contact the media producer or distributor directly, preferably by telephone, prior to order entry. Although such preorder communication with publishers is unusual in book and journal ordering, it may almost be considered the norm in acquisition of media materials. Given the generally high cost of purchasing and processing media materials, the potential cost of erroneously placed orders is significantly greater than the cost of a few long-distance telephone calls.

Table 5-1: Media Verification Sources

CD-ROM Products
CD-ROM Finder, 6th ed.
Kathleen Hogan and James Shelton, eds.Medford, NJ: Information Today, 1995.

CD-ROMs in Print (annual)
Westport, CT: Meckler.

"CD-ROMs in health sciences libraries"
Dudee Chiang. Med Ref Serv Q Summer 1993;12(2):67-81.

Gale Directory of Databases (annual)
Detroit, MI: Gale. (Vol 1: Online databases; vol. 2: CD ROM, etc.)

Computer Software
DATA Sources (semiannual)
New York: Ziff Communications.

Directory of Educational Software for Nursing, 5th ed.
Christine Boswell, ed. New York: National League for Nursing, 1993.

Healthcare CAI Directory (annual)
Scott Alan Stewart, ed. Alexandria, VA: Stewart Publishing.

 MD Computing Annual Directory of Medical Hardware and Software Companies (annual: July/August issue of *MD Computing*).
Secaucus, NJ: Springer Verlag.

Software Encyclopedia (annual).
New York: Reed Reference

Software for Health Sciences Education: A Resource Catalog, 6th ed.
Ann Arbor, MI: University of Michigan, 1995.

Internet Resources
Medical Matrix: Guide to Internet Clinical Medical Resources
http://www.slackinc.com/matrix

Directory of Electronic Journals and Newsletters.
Association of Research Libraries.
gopher://arl.cni.org:70/11/scomm/edir

Directory of Electronic Journals, Newsletters, and Academic Discussion Lists, 5th ed.
Washington, DC: Association of Research Libraries, 1995.

Videocassettes
Directory of Medical Video Programs
Charles M. Murtaugh, ed. Hawthorne, NJ: Ridge Publishing, 1990

The Video Source Book, 18th ed.
Christopher P. Scanlon, ed. Detroit: Gale Reserch, 1997.

Videodiscs
Healthcare Videodisc Directory (annual).
Scott Alan Stewart, ed. Alexandria, VA: Stewart Publishing.

In addition to confirming the identity, availability, and current price of items, the preorder telephone call can be used to review with the media publisher such items as previewing and special pricing policies. Information obtained by telephone should be fully documented — including the name of the individual providing the information — in the event that follow-up discussions are required. To avoid duplication of effort, it is also important that the media selector inform acquisitions personnel of any information already obtained from the publisher during the selection process.

Order Entry and Record-keeping

The actual mechanics of order entry, which generally involve transcription of the order information onto a multipart printed form or an automated acquisitions system order entry form, are more or less identical to those for print monographs and serials. A few additional points, however, need to be considered.

In designing or selecting a tracking system for media orders, be it manual or automated, consideration should be given to accommodating data elements unique to media items, such as format, version, and notes on handling of preview copies (e.g., preview period deadline, actual return date, previewer comments). Because media selectors frequently continue to be involved with the acquisitions process after order entry, they should ideally have direct and convenient access to online or printed order processing records.

The complexity of the media order (especially for digital items), combined with the fact that many media producers are relatively inexperienced in processing library orders, require that the order form itself be as clear and explicit as possible. Critical items, such as required format and whether or not a preview copy is required, should be highlighted.

Larger acquisitions operations may want to have a higher level supervisor do a final signoff on all media orders, or at least those with an estimated cost above a specified amount.

It is unusual for commercial media producers or distributors to require prepayment of institutional orders, and prepayment can be a hazardous gamble unless the reliability of the company is well established and the quality and suitability of the particular item is assured. A good, but by no means comprehensive, guide to producer and distributor policies on prepayment and other order requirements has been compiled by Pemberton [8].

Ordering Items on Preview

Although some media materials can only be purchased as firm orders, many media items are available on a preview or on-approval basis. There are many more factors involved in determining the suitability of a media item than there are for a book or journal, and many of these factors cannot be adequately determined without seeing or using the item in question. For example, librarians may want to try out the interface of a CD-ROM MEDLINE product and determine its ease of use before making a purchase decision. Similarly, a faculty member may want to view a videocassette to determine if the content is in accordance with the local curriculum, as well as determine the quality of the visuals.

Also, in most health sciences libraries, funding available for media acquisition is more limited than for other types of materials. Rather than acquiring several items on a specific topic that may provide a spectrum of viewpoints, the library usually purchases only one item that most closely matches local needs. Although the actual determination of which item to purchase falls within the purview of the selectors, acquiring the preview copies from which to make the decision is normally an acquisitions function.

Placing preview orders is similar to entering firm orders, except that the order itself must clearly specify the preview nature of the request. A standard form for preview requests simplifies the process. Unfortunately, the preview policies of the various media publishers differ, so it is the library's responsibility to determine individual policies either from publisher promotional material or by special inquiry. Some policies may be negotiable, including preview charges and the length of the preview period.

Once the preview item arrives in the library, it must be processed sufficiently for the program to be used by the evaluator (e.g., installed on a microcomputer or put into slide carousels), the evaluator contacted, the item reviewed, and a purchase decision made within the specified preview period. These steps in the preview process may be conducted by other departments, but the acquisition department should track the preview period to ensure that a purchase decision is made and the item returned if necessary in a timely manner. Extensions to preview periods can often be negotiated with the vendor. Care should be taken to ensure that return shipments are mailed and insured according to the publisher's instructions.

In cases where a decision is made to purchase the item on preview, several different procedures to finalize the purchase may ensue, depending again upon the policies of the particular publisher. Although some of these policies are documented in promotional material and catalogs, it is preferable to confirm these policies directly with the publisher at the time of order.

Often the cleanest procedure is to return the preview copy and enter a new firm order for the item. This procedure has the advantage of guaranteeing that the media copy obtained will be a new one, not one that has previously circulated as a preview copy. It has the disadvantage of requiring two separate order transactions, which can sometimes result in confusion or duplicate orders if not clearly documented. Alternatively, the library can keep the preview copy and request an invoice for the full purchase price. In this case, the preview order record must be updated to indicate that the order has been finalized.

Media publishers that do provide preview copies frequently assess a small preview charge for this service. Usually this charge is waived or subtracted from the purchase price if the item is retained. Some publishers do not officially offer a preview option, but do provide for purchase with "satisfaction guaranteed," which allows for items to be returned if not suitable within a specified period of time.

Receipt and Precataloging Processing of Media Orders

Once a media item has been received and, in the case of preview orders, the decision has been reached to add it to the collection, there is generally a need for a thorough precataloging review of the item by knowledgable acquisitions or media staff to determine that the item is complete and free of defects and to make decisions regarding library packaging, software installation parameters, handling of manuals, and special loan restrictions. This may also be the point at which a contents summary is written for inclusion in the cataloging record. Ideally all of these procedures should take place before the item is handled by the cataloging staff, since cataloging and holdings records for the item should reflect the local decisions made.

As with acquisition of other library materials, media items must first be checked to determine that the correct title and version have been received and that all the pieces are included. This process is considerably more complex than when a monograph arrives, since the media item is rarely a single physical item like a book. More typical are media titles consisting of a box of 35mm slides with an accompanying audiocassette and user's guide, or software packages with diskettes packaged with a manual and keyboard templates. The acquisitions department may do an initial screening to determine the completeness of the package or route it immediately to the requesting department or selector for a more thorough check before additional processing is performed.

Another step in receiving media materials is determining that the items are not defective. Since this assessment typically requires the item to be played on audiovisual equipment or installed on a computer, this evaluation is usually performed by staff of the media department. In any event, the item should be given at least a cursory examination (checking opening screen of a software program, spot checking sequences throughout a video- or audiocassette) as soon as possible to take advantage of limited return periods. Defective or mislabeled media items are a distressingly common occurrence. It is therefore prudent to build into the receiving process a thorough quality review.

Once the acquisitions staff has performed or delegated its responsibilities regarding the receipt of an item, they must ensure that the material is sent to the appropriate department involved in the further processing of the item. Since this may vary from item to item, the order request should indicate the routing of the item after check-in. A workform (Figure 5-1) indicating the steps that need to be performed and the department responsible is a useful device for ensuring that the item moves through the necessary procedures both before and after cataloging.

Fiscal Accounting

Although fiscal accounting for media purchases should be consistent with accounting practices for book and journal purchases, some additional procedures may need to be implemented to cope with the unique characteristics of media purchasing. First of all, careful consideration should be given to establishing useful and meaningful fund categories. Media purchases typically relate to a wide variety of library program areas, and it is useful if these can be closely reflected in fund allocation. At the very least, a clear differentiation should be made between materials purchased for staff use, such as general-purpose software titles, and materials purchased for patron use.

Separate fund categories should also be established for serial media titles, since these involve an ongoing committment of funds. If some media serials are handled by the library's subscription agency, it is helpful to have these titles billed in a special account so that charges for media serials can be tracked separately.

The high cost of individual media titles as well as the predominance of direct orders put a high premium on accuracy in entering and updating fiscal records. If a single book title is overlooked in calculating fund encumbrances, no great harm is done; if the same happens for a $2,500 software purchase, budget control can be seriously jeopardized. It is therefore prudent to perform additional checks on all media fiscal reports and to keep media selectors closely involved in the process.

Maintaining an accurate current picture of financial committments for media purchases is further complicated by the media previewing process.

[ ]Non-digital Media_______ [ ]Software

Title:

Date Initiated: __/__/__

Date Completed   Task

__/__/__ 1. Acquisitions/Serials - Receiving
    a. Receives item
    b. If preview material, note expiration date ___________ and go to step 3

__/__/__ 2. Cataloging - OCLC check.

__/__/__ 3. Learning Resources Center (LRC) - Clerical
    a. Checks in item.
    b. If AV media, go to step 6.

__/__/__ 4. LRC - Computer Consultant (for preview copies)
    a. If preview, verifies preview expiration date and records in software preview log.
    b. Tests software for reliability and usefulness.
    c. Gives recommendation to Media Librarian.

__/__/__ 5. LRC - Computer Consultant (for purchased copies)
    a. Installs and/or tests software for reliability.
    b. Takes print screen of opening menu.
    c. Photocopies diskette labels.
    d. Assembles manual, disks, printscreens, and photocopies.
    e. Sends in registration form
    f. Files copy of registration form

__/__/__ 6. LRC - Media Librarian
    a. Checks media for quality.
    b. Precatalogs and writes summary.

__/__/__ 7. LRC - Clerical
    a. Packages materials for shelving.
    b. Completes Cataloging form.

__/__/__ 8. Cataloging - Final processing
    a. Search OCLC if no previous copy found.
    b. Give to catalog librarian.
    c. OCLC input.
    d. Spine labeling and stamping.

__/__/__ 9. LRC - Clerical
    a. Special Labeling.
    b. If AV media, go to step 11.

__/__/__ 10. LRC - Computer Consultant
    a. Software made publicly available on network menu.
    b. Manuals routed to loan services IMMEDIATELY.

__/__/__ 11.Loan Services
    a. Places material on shelf for checkout.

Figure 5-1: Media Routing Form

Although funds for items ordered on preview have not actually been committed, it is useful for selectors and others to know the potential total cost of items currently in preview status. Therefore, the financial tracking system, whether manual or automated, must be capable of distinguishing between preview and firm-order purchases. Additionally, the preview fees themselves need to be counted as actual encumbrances, since they are payable even if the item is rejected.

Special Issues in Digital Media Acquisition

Licensing

The fundamental difference between most software purchases and other library acquisitions is that in the case of software the library is essentially purchasing a license to use the software, and its right to use the software is governed not only by the usual provisions of copyright law, but also by the terms of the license. Such terms typically require that the software not be altered, reproduced, or made available at more than one workstation without the consent of the producer and, in the case of networked availability, the payment of additional fees. Some licenses, such as those for many commerical software packages, are assumed to be in effect as soon as the purchaser unseals or installs the software; other licenses require the signature of an authorized library or institutional representative.

This license-based purchasing of digital media requires that some specialized procedures be in place for handling these materials.

- All licenses should be reviewed by a staff member responsible for ensuring library compliance with media licensing restrictions.

- Acquisitions staff should exercise caution in unpackaging commercial software, since this may involve implied acceptance of licensing restrictions.

- Procedures should be in place for payment of licensing fees, including possible annual fees and fees for multiple use. Normal acquisitions procedures may need to be considerably adjusted to accommodate "ordering" of—and payment for—legal permissions rather than physical objects.

- Licensing agreements are generally accompanied by some form of user registration system, which is also used to determine eligibility for free or discounted upgrades and for user support. A procedure should be in place for completing and returning registration forms and for keeping internal records on all currently registered software.

- Licensing terms may require that a product be returned if the licensing agreement is allowed to expire. Such returns should be carefully documented.

- For products such as CD-ROM databases, ongoing licensing fees may vary depending on how many years of indexing the library wants to retain.

Multiple-copy Licensing

In many institutional settings, it is desirable that a given software package or database product be available from more than one computer station and, in some cases, by more than one user at a time. This type of networked availability normally is permitted by producers only when a license for multiple use has been purchased. When multiple quantities are required for the library collection, directly contacting the publisher or vendor is usually required to determine the publisher's criteria for multiple use, as well as the pricing structure for additional stations or simultaneous users.

At the present time, there is little consistency among digital media producers regarding multiple-use licensing. Some publishers provide institutional site licenses after two copies at the regular price are purchased, others provide discounts if a minimum quantity are purchased or if groups of ten are purchased at one time. Negotiation of licensing terms may be a complicated and protracted process, requiring technical knowledge about the library's network environment and an understanding of anticipated usage levels [9].

Purchasing General-use Software

Purchasing commonly used software packages, such as those for word processing, spreadsheets, and presentation graphics, is often a perplexing task for acquisitions staff who may not be accustomed to the multiple distribution channels for these materials, including retail software stores and mail order wholesalers. Substantial differences in price and discounting policies can exist, so comparison shopping is worthwhile in this highly competitive market, especially when multiple copies are purchased. Large institutions may also have existing institution-wide contracts for discounted pricing with software publishers or vendors, requiring the library acquisitions staff to work closely with institutional purchasing agents.

This difficult area is made more confusing because general-use software usually accounts for only a small percentage of the library collection, and its purchase is therefore an uncommon event in the work of the acquisitions staff. For these reasons, some libraries that mainstream other types of media orders through the acquisitions department make an exception for general-use software, handling it instead through administrative or computer services departments.

Ordering Upgrades

Another acquisitions issue that arises with computer software is the handling of version upgrades. Almost all successful software products can be expected to evolve over a period of years through a succession of upgrades, which are generally offered to registered owners at reduced prices. This phenomenon first of all requires that when software arrives, registration cards be completed—typically by, and in the name of, the software selector—and returned to the publisher. Then, as new versions are available, the selector will be notified, allowing determination as to the necessity for upgrading to the newer version. These announcements specify the discounted pricing for upgrades, but usually require proof of ownership of an earlier version, such as the registration number or a serial number from the software.

As with the original purchase of the software product, pricing from various sources should be determined before purchasing an upgrade. In some cases, volume or educational discount pricing for software may be more attractive than the upgrade price, which is often not subject to volume or educational discounts. Upon receipt of software upgrades, acquisitions personnel should ensure that upgrades are routed through the cataloging department so that needed changes can be entered in bibliographic and holding records.

Maintenance and Customer-support Fees

A unique feature of the digital media purchase is that it may involve an ongoing payment of fees for customer support and maintenance. These fees are especially common for complex interactive products that are based on a large database of information requiring regular updating. In most cases these annual maintenance fees are less than the initial purchase price or license fee. For some programs, the maintenance fees may be tied to the licensing agreement and be required if the library wants to continue using the software; for some programs the fee pays for all software upgrades and updates of the information content.

Most maintenance agreements require the name of a single individual in the institution who is authorized to request user support and maintenance. When possible this invididual should be either the selector or the person most knowledgable about the particular piece of software. That individual will need to be consulted regularly to determine if renewal of the maintenance agreement is warranted.

CD-ROM Serials

Subscriptions to serially published media items, such as audio and video journals, as well as diskette- and CD-ROM-based journals and databases, often can be placed through regular library subscription agents. Placing these orders through a subscription agent provides the same advantages as it does for printed materials, e.g., simplified ordering, claiming, and payment processing. Although in the early days of CD-ROM serials, it was doubtful whether serials vendors were as knowledgable about the special problems of CD-ROM subscriptions as many librarians were, vendors have gained sophistication in their handling as more and more libraries have added these titles to their vendor-supplied lists. Service charges for these titles, however, should be closely monitored, since the high cost of some CD-ROM titles can result in exorbitant service charges when calculated on a percentage basis. Also, libraries should bear in mind that even if the title is handled by a vendor, the library may still need to deal directly with the publisher in such matters as negotiation of multiple-use charges and other special licensing terms [10].

Unlike most print serials subscriptions in which new issues are simply added to the file of previous issues, for many CD-ROM products new issues completely replace some or all of the earlier issues. For some titles, there may be considerable ambiguity about whether a new disk entirely supersedes the previous one; for these titles it is important that new disks be reviewed by professional staff who are completely familiar with the product.

A further complication in check-in of CD-ROM titles is that the subscription typically involves three different kinds of materials: 1) the compact disks themselves, 2) manuals and other documentation, including supplements or replacement pages, and 3) periodic upgrades to the search and display software, distributed either on diskette or CD-ROM. Each of these materials may require different types of routing and processing, involving staffs of the cataloging, automation, and public services staffs. It is therefore essential that the person performing check-in of these materials has clear instructions on how to identify and route each component of the subscription.

Network-distributed Publications

A growing number of publications—especially serials—in digital format are being distributed not in the form of microcomputer disks or CD-ROMs but rather as digital files distributed on the Internet [11-13]. Many electronic journals and newsletters automatically distribute the complete text of each issue to the e-mail addresses of subscribers; others distribute only a table of contents or brief summaries of the articles, along with instructions for requesting e-mail or FTP transmission of particular articles. Because effective cost recovery and access control mechanisms have not yet been standardized, most of these titles are distributed free of charge, and a large portion of them are government documents. This situation is likely to change as commercial publishers begin to grow more comfortable with electronic distribution.

Electronic serials look and behave very much like print serials and are amenable to many of the same acquisitions procedures. The major difference is that the issues arrive at a designated electronic mailbox rather than through the postal service. Libraries are currently in the process of working out the best procedure for checking in, routing, and storing electronic serial issues, and some generalized procedures are emerging [14-17].

- Issues are received at a designated electronic serials mailbox — in some cases a separate electronic mailbox for each title.

- Serials check-in staff record issues received in the regular serials check-in system.

- Issues are forwarded electronically to technical staff who strip out extraneous lines from the header of the e-mail message and store the issue as a file on a network-accessible server.

- Pointers to the files are created, typically using the menuing and searching capabilities provided in gopher, WAIS, World Wide Web, or similar software for network navigation.

In the future, it is expected that implementation of standards for title and issue identification in the header portion of each transmission may make it possible to fully automate most of the processing steps indicated above.

Of course, it is also possible to eliminate the first three steps above, and simply point the library's World Wide Web server to the publisher's or some other institution's Web site where the rest of the work has already been done. The end result from the library user's perspective is the same, although the only real "acquisition" activity that has taken place is the creation of an automatic link to the remote site and, in the case of nonpublic-domain materials, negotiation of and payment for the necessary permissions. In such cases, libraries need to decide whether and to what extent to include such titles in online catalogs and other holdings records. Indeed, such "acquisition by linkage" pushes the definition of "acquisition" to a point where it may cease to be a definable concept.

Commercial STM Journal Publishing in the Digital Era

The large, for-profit publishers of scientific journals are for the most part still in the experimental phase of finding viable electronic counterparts of their titles in print. Unlike the other network-distributed serials discussed in the preceding section, these electronic serials are being developed in a full graphical format, to accomodate complex illustrations and sophisticated gradations of font and type size. Some of these titles, such as the CD-ROM versions of *BMJ* and the *New England Journal of Medicine* from Maxwell Electronic Publishing, can be ordered and processed in the same way as the other CD-ROM serials discussed previously. However, raising more complex acquistions issues are new commercial ventures such as the ADONIS Document Delivery System and prototype projects, such as Elsevier's TULIP project and the Red Sage Project (involving primarily Springer-Verlag and Wiley titles in molecular biology and radiology)—all of which entail the licensing of access to established scientific journals in digital format [18-21]. The acquisitions challenge of these products is complicated by the fact that ongoing usage charges for printing or downloading of articles may be assessed.

Another model that is being tested for commercial publishing of scientific articles eliminates the concept of journal issues completely. Instead, articles are continuously added to a central database, which subscribers are authorized to search and selectively download. The innovator in implementing this approach has been the *Online Journal of Current Clinical Trials*, developed jointly by the American Association for the Advancement of Science and OCLC (and now a cooperative venture of OCLC and Chapman & Hall Publishers)[22-23]. Another journal distributed through the OCLC Electronic Journals Online Service is the *Online Journal of Knowledge Synthesis for Nursing.* Since additional connect time, downloading, and printing charges may be incurred, libraries may find that methods for handling these pay-as-you-go titles have more in common with interlibrary loan functions or with other database searching services than with standard serials acquisition procedures. In fact, it is in the handling of such titles that the much heralded merging of library acquisitions and document delivery operations may first become a reality.

Planning for the Future

Within the foreseeable future, a significant portion of library acquisitions will be in electronic format — and not simply text files or still graphics, but also full multimedia materials, including motion and sound. Many of these materials will not be amenable to existing acquisitions procedures for print books and journals, and many will not even involve the acquisition of a physical unit, but rather of legal access rights [24-25].

Libraries need to work to normalize the handling of these new materials in order to fulfill their basic function of making information available in a cost-effective manner. Until more standardized procedures are in place, acquisition of materials in new formats and with new licensing requirements will of necessity be a collaborative effort—involving the technical skills of computer experts, the planning and negotiating skills of administrators, the awareness of user needs of public services personnel, and the traditional organizational skills of library technical services staff [26]. The ability of libraries to rise to this challenge will to a great extent determine their relevance and usefulness in the coming decade and beyond [27].

References

1. Cummings AM, Witte ML, Bowen WG, Lazarus LO, et al. University libraries and scholarly communication: a study prepared for The Andrew W. Mellon Foundation. Chicago: Association of Research Libraries, 1992.

2. LaPorte RE, Marler E, Akazawa S, Sauer F, et al. The death of biomedical journals. BMJ 1995 May 27;310(6991):1387-90.

3. Bosch S, Promis P, Sugnet C. Guide to selecting and acquiring CD-ROMs, software, and other electronic publications. Chicago: American Library Association, 1994. (Acquisition guidelines no. 7).

4. Atkinson R. The acquisitions librarian as a change agent in the transition to the electronic library. Lib Res Tech Serv 1992 Jan; 36(1):7-20.

5. Chiang K, Curtis H. The selection and acquisition of software and computerized data. In: Curtis C, ed. Public access microcomputers in academic libraries: the Mann Library model at Cornell University. Chicago: American Library Association, 1987:49-58.

6. Hayes JM. Acquiring special formats. In: Schmidt KA, ed. Understanding the business of library acquisitions. Chicago: American Library Association, 1990:239-257.

7. Mircheff JG. Resources for health sciences educational software. Med Ref Serv Q 1993 Winter; 12(4):45-50.

8. Pemberton JM. Policies of audiovisual producers and distributors: a handbook for acquisitions personnel. 2nd ed. Metuchen, NJ: Scarecrow, 1989.

9. Nissley M, Nelson NM, eds. CD-ROM licensing and copyright issues for librarians. Westport CT: Meckler, 1990.

10. Davis TL. Acquisition of CD-ROM databases for local area networks. J Acad Libr 1993 May;19(2):68-71.

11. Bailey CW. Network-based electronic serials. Info Tech Libs 1992 March; 11(1):29-35.

12. Sasse M, Winkler BJ. Electronic journals: a formidable challenge for libraries. Adv Libr 1993; 17:149-73.

13. Okerson A, O'Donnell J, eds. Scholarly journals at the crossroads: a subversive proposal for electronic publishing. Washington, DC: Association of Research Libraries, 1995.

14. Parang E, Saunders L. Electronic journals in ARL libraries: policies and procedures. Washington, DC: Association of Research Libraries, 1994. (SPEC Kit no. 201).

15. Parang E, Saunders L. Electronic journals in ARL libraries: issues and trends. Washington, DC: Association of Research Libraries, 1994. (SPEC Kit no. 202).

16. Manoff M, Brandt DS, Snowden C, Zuppel C, et al. MIT libraries electronic journals project: report on patron access and technical processing. Ser Rev 1993 Fall; 19(3):15-40.

17. Keating LR, Reinke CE, Goodman JA. Electronic journal subscriptions. Libr Acquis Pract Theory 1993 Winter; 17(4):455-63.

18. Leach RG, Tribble JE. Electronic document delivery: new options for libraries. J Acad Librarianship 1993 Jan; 18(6);359-365.

19. Butter K. Red Sage: the next step in delivery of electronic journals. Med Ref Serv Q 1994 Fall; 13(3):75-81.

20. Hoffman MM, O'Gorman L, Story GA, Arnold JQ, et al. The RightPages service: an image-based electronic library. J Am Soc Info Sci 1993 Sep; 44(8):446-452.

21. Borman S. Advances in electronic publishing herald changes for scientists. Chem Eng News 1993 Jun 14; :10-24.

22. Keyhani A. The Online Journal of Current Clinical Trials: an innovation in electronic journal publishing. Database 1993 Feb;16(1):14-15,17-20,22-23.

23. Brahmi FA, Kaneshiro K. The Online Journal of Current Clinical Trials (OJCCT): a closer look. Med Ref Serv Q 1993 Fall; 12(3):29-43.

24. Garrett JR. Digital libraries: the grand challenges. EDUCOM Rev 1993 July/Aug;28(4):17-21.

25. Odlyzko AM. Tragic loss or good riddance? The impending demise of traditional scholarly journals. Surfaces [electronic journal] 1994;4 (105). gopher://surfaces.umontreal.ca.

26. Braude RM, Florance V, Frisse M, Fuller S. The organization of the digital library. Acad Med 1995 April;70(4):286-91.

27. Graham PS. Requirements for the digital research library. Coll Res Libr 1995 July;56(4):331-39.

Glossary

AAAS	American Association for the Advancement of Science
ABLE	Advanced bindery/library exchange
ACQNET	Electronic newsletter on acquisitions for academic librarians.
ACQWEB	World Wide Web site affiliated with ACQNET
AHEC	Area Health Education Center
AICPA	American Institute of Certified Public Accountants
ALA	American Library Association
ALCTS	Association for Library Collections and Technical Services (ALA)
AMA	American Medical Association
ANSI	American National Standards Institute
ANSI ASC	ANSI Accredited Standards Committee
AVIAC	Automation Vendor Information and Advisory Committee (ALA)
AVLINE	Audiovisuals Online (database—NLM)
BIP	*Books in Print*
BISAC	Book Industry Systems Advisory Committee
BITNET	Because It's Time Network
BLAB	Biomedical Library Acquisitions Bulletin (electronic newsletter)
CATLINE	Cataloging Online (database—NLM)
CD-ROM	Compact Disc, Read-Only Memory
CIOMS	Council for International Organizations of Medical Sciences
CIP	Cataloging in publication
CMBLS	Checklist of Microcomputer Based Library Software
COM	Computer output microform
CONSER	Cooperative Online Serials (LC)
DIALOG	Online search service (Dialog Information Services, Inc.)
DOCLINE	Documents Online (NLM)

EDI	Electronic data interchange
EDIFACT	EDI for Administration, Commerce, and Transport
FASB	Financial Accounting Standards Board
FAX	Telefacsimile
FEIN	Federal Employer Identification Number
FTP	File transfer protocol
GPO	Government Printing Office (U.S.)
IARC	International Agency for Research on Cancer
ILL	Interlibrary loan
ILS	Integrated library system
INTERLOC	Online database of out-of-print books
Internet	Network of networks using standard telecommunications software
ISBN	International Standard Book Number
ISO	International Organization for Standardization
ISSN	International Standard Serials Number
LAN	Local Area Network
LBI	Library Binding Institute
LC	Library of Congress
MARC	Machine Readable Cataloging
MEDLARS	MEDical Literature Analysis and Retrieval System (database—NLM)
MEDLINE	MEDLARS Online (database—NLM)
MeSH	Medical Subject Headings
MISHULS	Michigan Statewide Health Sciences Union List of Serials
MLA	Medical Library Association
NASIG	North American Serials Interest Group
NISO	National Information Standards Organization
NLM	National Library of Medicine
NLN	National League for Nursing
NN/LM	National Network of Libraries of Medicine
NSDP	National Serials Data Program (LC)
NTIS	National Technical Information Service
OCLC	Online Computer Library Center
OP	Out-of-print
OPAC	Online Public Access Catalog

ORBIT	Online Retrieval of Bibliographic Information Timeshared
PAHO	Pan American Health Organization
PIIRC	Publishing and Information Industries Relations Committee (MLA)
RFP	Request for proposals
RFQ	Request for quotations
RLIN	Research Libraries Information Network
SERHOLD	Serials Holdings Online (database - NLM)
SERLINE	Serials Online (database—NLM)
SISAC	Serials Industry Systems Advisory Committee
SICI	Serial Item and Contributor Identifier
STM	Science, Technology, Medicine (international group of publishers)
STN	Scientific and Technical Information Network
SuDoc	Superintendent of Documents (U.S.)
USBE	United States Book Exchange
VHS	Video Home System
WAIS	Wide Area Information Service
WHO	World Health Organization
WLN	Washington Library Network
WWW	World Wide Web
X12	Standardized electronic ordering format (Accredited Standards Committee X12 of ANSI)
Z39	Bibliographic standards for storing and retrieving information (ANSI)

Index

This is primarily a subject index. Personal authors of references cited in the text are not indexed. Acronyms and initialisms are given preference as indexing terms if more commonly used than full names of organizations or publications.

Author Biographies

Janis F. Brown has been the Associate Director for Educational Resources at the Norris Medical Library at the University of Southern California for the past nine years. Since 1983, she has been responsible for the library's media and microcomputer facilities and services including acquiring appropriate materials and making them available to users. She has also been involved in Internet Gopher and World Wide Web server developments at USC, including providing electronic journals both locally and through connections to Internet resources.

Barbara A. Carlson is a health sciences librarian whose work experience with serials dates from 1972 and specifically within the medical library arena since 1980. Actively involved in serials professional issues, she integrates her interests and activities with those of publishers, subscription agencies, binders, systems developers, other librarian specialists, and library users. Formerly the Head of Serials Management at the Medical University of South Carolina, she is now Coordinator of Consumer Information and Education and holds the MUSC faculty rank of Associate Professor.

Mark E. Funk is Head of Collection Development at Cornell University Medical Library in New York City. He has been a health sciences librarian since 1976 and has managed collection development, serials, and acquisitions since 1980. A founding member of MLA's Library Research Section, he has published papers on indexing consistency in MEDLINE and on the usefulness of monographic proceedings.

Daniel H. Jones is Assistant Library Director for Collection Development at the Briscoe Library of the University of Texas Health Science Center at San Antonio. He has worked in medical libraries since 1977. He serves on the editorial board of *Serials Review* and the *Newsletter on Serials Pricing Issues*, and is a member of the Springer-Verlag Library Advisory Council. He has been an active member of the North American Serials Interest Group (NASIG), having served on several ad hoc and standing committees, and as the MLA liaison to NASIG.

David H. Morse has been actively involved in technical services and collection development since 1976, first at the Philadelphia College of Pharmacy and Science and then at the University of Southern California Norris Medical Library. At USC he developed the microcomputer-based CATS acquisitions system, and he is the founding editor of the *Biomedical Library Acquisitions Bulletin,* the electronic newsletter of the Collection Development Section of the Medical Library Association. With Daniel Richards he compiled the MLA Doc Kit *Collection Development Policies for Health Sciences Libraries* (MLA, 1992).

Pat L. Walter spent over 30 years affiliated with the Louise M. Darling Biomedical Library at UCLA, the last thirteen as Associate Biomedical Librarian for Technical Services, overseeing Collection Development, Acquisitions, and Cataloging; for the last two years she also assumed direct responsibility for collection development. She retired from the University in 1994. Her MLA contributions include serving as Proceedings Editor and Associate Editor of the *Bulletin of the Medical Library Association* and Section Council representative for the Medical Informatics Section. She is a member of the Literature Selection Technical Review Committee of the National Library of Medicine.

Judith C. Wilkerson is a medical librarian with experience in reference and document delivery in addition to serials. As an Information Sciences Intern at the National Cancer Institute, as Head of Serials at the University of Texas Southwestern Medical Center at Dallas Library, and in her current position she has participated in planning and implementation of transitions between serials management systems. She has helped organize a statewide serials interest group for academic libraries in Oklahoma and has chaired the Serials Subcommittee of the Association for Higher Education of North Texas. She is currently Assistant Professor of Medical Library Science at the University of Oklahoma Health Sciences Center where she is Head of Serials Services at the Robert M. Bird Health Sciences Library.